Progress in Clinical Neurologic Trials
Volume 1

Amyotrophic Lateral Sclerosis

Progress in Clinical Neurologic Trials

Vol. 1: *Amyotrophic Lateral Sclerosis,* edited by F. Clifford Rose, M.D.

Vol. 2: *Parkinson's Disease,* edited by F. Clifford Rose, M.D.

PROGRESS IN CLINICAL NEUROLOGIC TRIALS

Volume 1

Amyotrophic Lateral Sclerosis

EDITOR

F. Clifford Rose, M.D.

Director, Academic Unit of Neuroscience
Charing Cross and Westminster Medical School
University of London
and
Physician-in-Charge
Department of Neurology
Regional Neurosciences Centre
Charing Cross Hospital
London, England

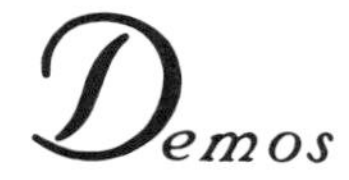

Demos Publications, 156 Fifth Avenue, New York, New York 10010

Made in the United States of America

Great care has been taken to maintain the accuracy of the information contained in this volume. However, neither the editor nor Demos Publications can be held responsible for errors or for any consequences arising from the use of the information contained herein.

ISBN: 0-939-957-23-X
LC: 89-081930

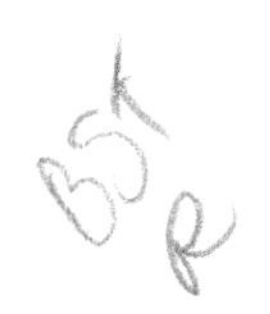

Series Foreword

This is the first in a series of monographs on methodological problems in clinical trials of neurological disorders. An underlying premise to the development of such a series is that each neurological disorder requires different protocols. For example, diagnostic certainty is high in amyotrophic lateral sclerosis (ALS), but less so in multiple sclerosis (MS), of which most classifications divide cases into definite, probable, and possible, and even less so in migraine, where there is no laboratory marker.

The course of each disease varies, from the invariably progressive course of ALS through the remitting nature of MS to such disorders as migraine, in which cases can vary enormously with regard to frequency of attacks and the disability caused.

Since the majority of clinicians are not involved in clinical trials, why should they know about their methodological problems? The answer is to understand and assess therapeutic claims that are made. The history of many neurological disorders is replete with treatments claimed to be effective, raising hopes falsely with consequent ill effects on patients and their caretakers. There is only one way to scientifically prove that treatment works and that is by clinical trials, the science of experimental epidemiology. The problems lie in their methodological difficulties, be they poor selection, too few numbers of patients, or a host of other traps into which the unwary may fall. Some of these traps are revealed in the following pages and the volumes to come in this series.

To perform unsound clinical trials is a waste of time for patients and health-care workers, and a waste of money in the health-care field, where universally hard-pressed financial conditions also make unsound clinical trials unethical.

If such problems can be avoided in the future, the efforts of the contributors to this series will not be wasted.

F. Clifford Rose, M.D.

Preface

Why should clinical therapeutic trials be necessary for a disease such as amyotrophic lateral sclerosis (ALS), with its invariably progressive course and fatal end? One authority has stated that, if a cure could be found, then only five patients would be necessary to establish its value. Unfortunately, a cure, in the sense of completely stopping disease progression, is unlikely, and even more remote is the recovery of neurons of the central nervous system that have been damaged. The more probable scenario is the discovery of a drug that could retard the disease's progression, and it is here that the problems of assessment arise.

The assessment of motor power is not easy, since there are so many variables, not least in the patient and his environment, so that objective methods are required. Although the course of the disease is always progressive, the rate of deterioration will vary in each patient, although the slope of this decline remains the same in each patient. This applies to the death and fallout of neurons but may not be seen clinically because of such variables as cooperation, fatigue, and assessment methods.

The history of drugs that have been claimed to be effective in ALS is full of false hopes, but there is no doubt that the science of experimental neuroepidemiology has improved in recent years. From the type of drugs used can be traced the fashionable etiological theories of the time, e.g., in the 1970s, when ALS was considered to be immunological, immunosuppressants such as cortisone, immunostimulants such as levamisole, or immune factors such as transfer factor or thymic factor were used. When the viral theory was in the ascendant, amantadine, interferon, and cytoarabinase C were tried. More recently, gangliosides and amino acids such as *N*-acetylcysteine, l-threonine, and branched-chain amino acids have been given but without the proof of methodologically sound clinical trials.

The cure has not yet come, but the search continues. When a possible cure presents itself, it will behoove us to be ready to have the proper methods to prove its efficacy. This volume is an attempt to establish these methods to advance the progress of these studies.

This book should be of value not only to those attempting to perform clinical trials but also to those who need to assess therapeutic claims. This will therefore include all those dealing with patients suffering from this awesome condition, not only neurologists and neuroscientists but all doctors, paramedics, and caretakers who are entrusted with the care of those whose only hope is that an effective treatment will be found in their much-shortened life span. As the title of the first chapter suggests, that hope is greater in this recombinant era.

F. Clifford Rose, M.D.

Contents

Contributors

Patricia Andres, R.P.T., M.S., Neuromuscular Research Unit and MDA/ALS Treatment and Research Center, Tufts – New England Medical Center, Boston, Massachusetts, U.S.A.

A. S. Brooke, B.Sc., M.C.S.P., Academic Unit of Neuroscience, Charing Cross and Westminster Medical School, London, England.

Sebastian Conradi, M.D., Department of Neurology, Karolinska Sjukuset, Stockholm, Sweden.

Paul De Koning, M.D., Department of Neurology, University of Utrecht, Utrecht, The Netherlands.

Eric H. Denys, M.D., ALS and Neuromuscular Research Center, Pacific Presbyterian Medical Center, San Francisco, California, U.S.A.

P. M. Enderby, Ph.D., FCST, Department of Neurology, University of Bristol, Frenchay Hospital, Bristol, England.

Barry W. Festoff, M.D., Professor, Department of Neurology, University of Kansas Medical Center; and Medical Investigator of the Veterans Administration, Kansas City, Missouri, U.S.A.

James Frane, Ph.D., Genentech Corporation, San Francisco, California, U.S.A.

Mark R. Glasberg, M.D., Department of Neurology, Henry Ford Hospital, Detroit, Michigan, U.S.A.

R. J. Guiloff, M.D., FRCP, Consultant Neurologist and Honorary Senior Lecturer, Department of Neurology, Westminster Hospital, Charing Cross and Westminster Medical School, London, England.

R. Langton Hewer, M.D., FRCP, Consultant Neurologist, Bristol; and Clinical Lecturer, Department of Neurology, University of Bristol, Frenchay Hospital, Bristol, England.

Allen D. Hillel, M.D., Associate Professor, Otolaryngology/Head and Neck Surgery, University of Washington; and Chief, Otolaryngology/Head and Neck Surgery, Seattle Veterans Affairs Medical Center, Seattle, Washington, U.S.A.

Masao Honda, M.D., Director, Department of Neurology, Yokohama City Hospitals, Yokohama, Japan.

David A. Ingram, M.D., Section of Neurological Sciences, The London Hospital, Whitechapel, London, England.

Sherri Jacoby, R.N., Center for Neurologic Study, San Diego, California, U.S.A.

Frans G. I. Jennekens, M.D., Department of Neurology, University of Utrecht, Utrecht, The Netherlands.

Catherine Jones, MCST, Speech Therapist, Charing Cross Hospital, London, England.

Nancy Konikow, R.N., M.N., CNRN, Neurological Clinical Nurse, Neurology Service, University Hospital; and Specialist Clinical Assistant Professor, Department of Physiological Nursing, University of Washington, Seattle, Washington, U.S.A.

Gerald Kuether, M.D., Department of Neurology, Technical University of Munich, Neurologische Klinik und Poliklinik, Munich, F.R.G.

Russell J. M. Lane, BSc, M.D., MRCP, Consultant Neurologist, Regional Neurosciences Centre, Charing Cross Hospital, London, England.

Hans Gerd Lipinski, Ph.D., Department of Neurology, University of Munich, Neurologische Klinik und Poloklinik, Munich, F.R.G.

Elisabeth S. Louwerse, M.D., Department of Neurology, University of Amsterdam, Academisch Medisch Centrum, Amsterdam, The Netherlands.

Evelyn McDonald, M.S., Director, ALS Patient Project, New Road Map Foundation, Seattle, Washington, U.S.A.

Schlomo Melmed, M.D., Cedar Sinai Hospital, Los Angeles, California, U.S.A.

Robert M. Miller, Ph.D., Clinical Assistant Professor, Speech and Hearing Sciences, Rehabilitation Medicine, and Otolaryngology/Head and Neck Surgery, University of Washington; and Chief, Audiology and Speech Pathology Service, Seattle Veterans Affairs Medical Center, Seattle, Washington, U.S.A.

H. Modarres-Sadeghi, M.D., MRCP, Research Fellow, Department of Neurology, Westminster Hospital, London, England.

Gabriella Molnari, Ph.D., Cedar Sinai Hospital, Los Angeles, California, U.S.A.

Theodore L. Munsat, M.D., Professor of Neurology and Pharmacology, Tufts - New England Medical Center, Boston, Massachusetts, U.S.A.

Forbes H. Norris, M.D., Vice-President and Clinical Director, ALS and Neuromuscular Research Foundation; and Neurologist, Pacific Presbyterian Medical Center, San Francisco, California, U.S.A.

Lori Peterson, B.A., Kansas City Veterans Administration Medical Center, Kansas City, Missouri, U.S.A.

Paolo Pinelli, M.D., Professor of Nervous and Mental Diseases and Full Professor of Neurology, Biomedical Sciences, St. Paolo Teaching Hospital, University of Milan, Milan, Italy.

Fabrizio Pisano, M.D., Department of Neurology, Medical Center of Rehabilitation, Clinica del Lavoro Foundation, Institute of Care and Research, Veruno, Italy.

I. C. Robinson, Ph.D., John Bevan Research Unit, Department of Human Sciences, Brunel, The University of West London, London, England.

H. Rogers, Senior Physiological Measurement Technician, Department of Neurology, Westminster Hospital, London, England.

Lars-Olof Ronnevi, M.D., Department of Clinical Neurology, Karolinska Sjukhuset, Stockholm, Sweden.

Barry Sherman, M.D., Genentech Corporation, San Francisco, California, U.S.A.

Linda Skerry, A.S., Neuromuscular Research Unit and MDA/ALS Treatment and Research Center, Tufts-New England Medical Center, Boston, Massachusetts, U.S.A.

Richard Alan Smith, M.D., Center for Neurologic Study, San Diego, California, U.S.A.

T. J. Steiner, M.B., Ph.D., Academic Unit of Neuroscience, Charing Cross and Westminster Medical School, London, England.

Yolanda van der Graff, M.D., Department of Public Health and Epidemiology, University of Utrecht, Utrecht, The Netherlands.

J. M. B. Vianney de Jong, M.D., Department of Neurology, University of Amsterdam, Academisch Medisch Centrum, Amsterdam, The Netherlands.

George H. Wieneke, Ph.D., Department of Clinical Neurophysiology, University of Utrecht, Utrecht, The Netherlands.

Kathryn Yorkston, Ph.D., Professor, Department of Rehabilitation Medicine, University of Washington, Seattle, Washington, U.S.A.

Amyotrophic Lateral Sclerosis,
edited by F. Clifford Rose.
Demos Publications, New York © 1990.

1

ALS Clinical Trials: Hope in the Recombinant Era

Barry W. Festoff

Neurobiology Research Laboratory, Kansas City Veterans Administration Medical Center, and Department of Neurology, University of Kansas Medical Center, Kansas City, MO, U.S.A.

Twelve years ago, I was asked by the organizing committee of a meeting on amyotrophic lateral sclerosis (ALS), sponsored by the ALS Society of America and chaired by Dr. Donald Mulder, to review the world's literature on ALS and motor neuron disease (ALS.MND) clinical trials. A literature search had already been initiated by Dr. Thomas Chase, NINCDS, NIH, and his colleagues and that was given to me. I then engaged the assistance of our ALS nurse-clinician from the University of Kansas Medical Center, Nancy Jones-Crigger, and we began our adventure. After some 10 months, we had completed our travail and produced a chapter for the proceedings of that meeting, held in Tucson, Arizona, and edited by Dr. Mulder (1). It was not a particularly pleasant, or even hopeful, experience. We developed criteria for evaluating the 800-odd reports of "clinical trials" in ALS.MND (2) and discovered, much to our dismay and consternation, that all published ALS.MND treatment trials, save for one or two, failed to meet the criteria we had established (2).

Much has happened over the last 10 years to change that dismal outlook. To be sure, the cure for ALS.MND has not yet been discovered, in spite of optimism over recent candidates such as thyrotropin releasing hormone (TRH) (3–6). Likewise the cause(s) of ALS.MND have not been determined, although some recent proposals have been getting considerable attention (7–20). Over this same period, there has been no real shortage of meetings devoted to issues in ALS.MND clinical and basic research(1,21–24), but this volume represents the published proceedings of a meeting that took place in June 1988 at the Charing Cross Hospital, London, which was unique compared to the other symposia. It was *entirely devoted* to considerations of the methodological problems underlying ALS.MND therapeutic trials. Such a

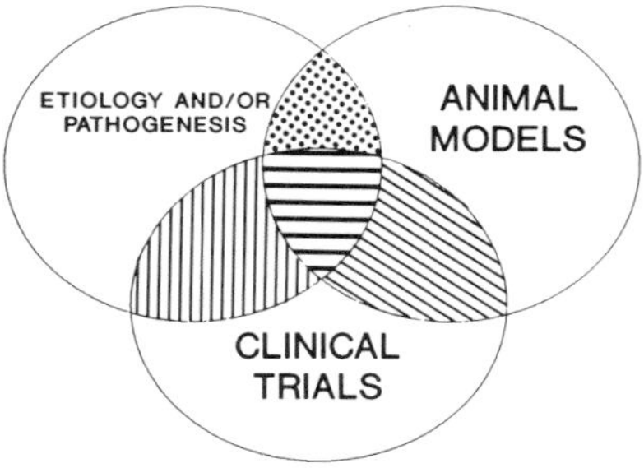

FIG. 1-1. Three-ring sign of research in ALS.MND.

topic was really unheard of, even unthought of, a decade ago. Over this same time period, the modern biological revolution of growth/trophic factors, monoclonal antibody production, molecular biology, and reverse molecular genetics has also taken place and is still evolving. The advent of the modern clinical trial methodology has advanced, initiated by traditional journals as well as those concerned primarily with the issues of trial design and conduct (e.g., *Journal of Clinical Trials*). These concurrent events are certain to have a positive impact on ALS.MND trials in the future.

This chapter represents not so much an introduction but a chronicle of a brighter future for ALS.MND clinical trial research, which must continue in parallel and be integrated with basic and clinical research (Fig.1-1) along with provision of state-of-the-art services for ALS.MND patients. It is important to concentrate on recent successes in clinical trial design and methodological concepts of conducting such trials with ALS.MND patients. Thus, the meeting at Charing Cross represented a unique experience for all who participated in it and a historic milestone in the almost 140-year history of medical awareness of ALS.MND (25–27). The meeting was not totally harmonious and, in fact, debate was, at times heated, and time did not allow for the publication of a "white paper" or set of accords.

However, a generally positive spirit emerged from this meeting, which must be credited to the international flavor, largely emanating from the ALS.MND Research Foundation, directed by William Parlette, and its Scientific Advisory Committee, chaired by F. Clifford Rose. Initiated at the Kyoto meeting, organized by Dr. Yoshiro Yase and the late Dr. Tadao Tsubaki, the Scientific Advisory Committee of the ALS.MND Research Foundation agreed to hold workshops every 6 months dealing with critical issues in research of ALS.MND. This meeting in London concerning methodological problems in the conduct of ALS.MND clinical trials represents the first of these workshops.

Although a "white paper" was not produced at the conclusion of the meeting, considerable consensus developed along the lines of what was needed for the future, and even "agreements to disagree" resulted, which allowed for the possibility of fruitful collaborations in the future. One important outcome was the formation of subcommittees to develop approaches for the standardization of future clinical trials in ALS.MND. Reports of the subcommittee chairpersons will be presented at future workshops and summarized in *Update,* the quarterly issue of the ALS.MND Research Foundation, and distributed as widely as possible to investigators and clinicians as well as lay groups in the field.

In this chapter, those presentations at the London meeting in which developments were considered to be the most productive in future ALS.MND trial design are summarized.

NOMENCLATURE, PATIENT SELECTION, AND STRATIFICATION

Critical in the earlier review was the difficulty in determining the condition being evaluated and treated with an experimental therapy (2). This is extended to the controversy concerning the four major types of adult, sporadic MND: "classic" ALS, progressive bulbar palsy (PBP), progressive muscular atrophy (PMA), and primary lateral sclerosis (PLS). Conradi (Chapter 2) discusses the nosology and nomenclature, comparing the inexactness of the British term, MND, and the French/U.S./Japanese term, ALS, and shows the double meaning and confusion arising out of both terms. He concluded that early diagnosis was essential, but, as pointed out earlier by Munsat and Bradley (28), as many as 7–10% of patients with "classic" ALS may only have lower motor neuron (LMN) involvement early in the course of the illness, an important factor in stratification of patients, as discussed by Guiloff et al. (Chapter 3). Some groups

be syndromic with multifactorial etiology, perhaps with a common pathogenetic mechanism (2,7,8,21–24,28). Included in this category of considerations are inclusion and exclusion criteria (7,8,28). Disease stage is an issue for both underlying cause(s) as well as for therapeutic trial considerations, where maximal efficacy must be a prime concern. Although a consensus was not reached in this area, patient selection is discussed by Glasberg (Chapter 4).

WHAT TO MEASURE

Muscle Strength

As was shown by numerous studies of victims of the poliomyelitis epidemics, as reviewed by Lane (Chapter 7), functional muscle testing lags behind manual muscle testing. Manual muscle testing (when performed by a specially trained registered physical therapist), as has been shown in studies of Duchenne muscular dystrophy obligate carriers (29), predicts weakness that is not clearly detected functionally, bringing in the concept of *clinimetrics,* as conceived by Feinstein (30). The relationship between power, on an ordinal scale, and number of remaining functional motor neurons is a major area for discussion, that is, scales versus interval measurements. In terms of strength measurements, it is important to decide on isometric or isokinetic systems. For instance, there are better correlations of leg isometric strength and the "Norris scale" (31) or "Appel scale" (28) than there are for arm measurements, but this is reversed for isokinetic measures, in which arm correlates with Norris ALS disability scores better than leg (Chapter 10). Discussions of torque, rather than simple strength, further the thinking on this important issue. Exercise capacity, used by Brooks and his colleagues at the University of Wisconsin, was also introduced. Dr. Theodore Munsat, who also chaired this session, reviewed his experience with the Tufts Quantitative Neuromuscular Examination or TQNE (32). His additional information, based on a six-factor rotated factor analysis, suggested classic ALS is a regional disease (in that bulbar problems occur quite late in some patients) and that, because of the linearity of disease progression, patients might serve as their own historical controls (Chapter 8). Such information, if confirmed, would allow for rapid small-scale, single-center, open trials to test candidate agents.

Bulbar Function: Dysarthria and Dysphagia

In none of the proposed measuring instruments, neither scales nor interval measures, are deficits in bulbar function adequately handled. At the meeting, Catherine Jones of the Charing Cross Hospital Dysphagia Unit (Chapter 13), discussed a recent pilot study designed to measure changes in bulbar function in 20 ALS.MND patients (13 men and 7 women). Only 11 of the patients had a bulbar onset of their disease. They studied swallowing, using liquid (250%, w/v, barium), semi-solid (blancmange), and solid (a tea biscuit) media and divided swallowing into oral, oropharyngeal, and esophageal phases. Of interest, the tongue was most abnormal, with pharyngeal function next, followed by abnormal trigger, aspiration, lip, and then, soft-palate weakness, and finally, cricopharyngeal spasticity. Radiologically, the soft palate and pharynx were most reliable indices, suggesting that these may be easily organized for clinical trial follow-up. Speech therapy may be a predictor of aspiration, on a statistical basis, and this is both an important clinical point as well as a possible quantitative measure for therapeutic trials. Some confirmation of this point came from Dr. A. Hillel (Chapter 11), who presented an ordinal disability scale for ALS.MND patients. He showed that forced vital capacity (FVC) and phonation correlated well with state of disability: greater than 10 s correlated with FVC under 1 L. He also showed an overall reliability coefficient of 0.95, highest with speaking and swallowing (r = 0.81) and lowest for upper and lower extremity strength (r = 0.59). When bulbar function and extremity strength were compared, the correlation coefficient was extremely low. He concluded that such an ALS severity scale was suitable for open trials and is planning such a trial in the near future.

NEW ASSESSMENT METHODS

In this area, the work of Dr. T. Zephiro (unpublished observations) may be applicable to ALS.MND, at least early in the course of patients with upper motor neuron (UMN) greater than LMN disability. He utilized a digital tablet with lighted targets to assess variability of movement. Using such a system he has already determined that visual integration of movement was impaired in patients with Parkinson's disease. Drs. Eric Denys, San Francisco (Chapter 15), critically evaluated the usefulness of electromyography (EMG) in ALS.MND clinical trials and concluded that most EMG studies were of limited value in following the course of ALS.MND. However, Drs. Jennekens and De Koning in Utrecht (Chapter 17) have set up a clinical trial to study the effects of one candidate agent, a synthetic peptide, ORG 2766 (amino acids 4–9), on correlates of reinnervation in muscle of patients with ALS.MND. They will study jitter and fiber density, as well as motor unit size, which are all increased, in ALS.MND. The agent, which is similar to a peptide in *alpha* MSH/ACTH, appears to positively influence nerve regeneration in denervated muscle.

Dr. D. Ingram in London (Chapter 16) has been using a magnetic stimulator to estimate central motor conduction time (CMCT) in ALS.MND patients, in the hope of obtaining a quantitative measurement that could be followed in therapeutic trials. One question that was raised was whether it was possible to stimulate either corticospinal tract separately, important in that it would be theoretically possible that the normal CMCT might cancel out the abnormal, possibly even midway. Ingram suggested that right and left corticospinal tracts could be separated by this technique. He further showed that the greater CMCT correlated with extensor plantar responses clinically. Such a magnetic stimulator carries a current price tag of $20,000.

Potentially very important in the planning of ALS.MND experimental trials is computer modeling data (Kuether and Lipinski, Chapter 21). They have approached this problem by using a Monte Carlo simulation of LMN disease as might be found in PMA or early in a patient with classic ALS who has not developed UMN symptoms. Of interest was the finding that the amount of preserved force in the computer model was not directly correlated with the percentage of motor neuron loss, which may contradict empirical data obtained from TQNE (32). From this modeling study it appeared that reinnervated muscle fibers, and reinnervation is very prominent in ALS.MND (33), do not retain the original strength or force prior to denervation. In fact, with the last 5% of remaining motor neurons there is no efficient reinnervation. Thus, the reinnervation potential falls off with progressive loss of motor neurons despite the fact that in some ALS.MND patients the efficiency of reinnervation, and subsequent force development, is quite good for some time.

SCALES OR INTERVAL MEASURES OF MOTOR NEURONS

The most heated debate centers on whether to utilize traditional reliance on scales, such as the Norris (31) and Appel scales (28), or to concentrate on exploring further interval measures such as the TQNE (32). A scale being used now at the University of Washington (Hillel et al., Chapter 11) has some of the qualities of both systems, and should prove useful, at least for open trials. Another scale (Honda, Chapter 9) may have utility in the respiratory area, since the ratio of minimal divided by maximal chest circumference

$$\text{Ratio } (\%) = \frac{\text{Chest circum}_{\text{min}}}{\text{Chest circum}_{\text{max}}}$$

is an indicator of respiratory muscle capacity.

BIOSTATISTICS AND DATABASES

The central limit theorem (34) states that with large enough sample sizes the sum of observations from any distribution is approximately normally distributed. Consequently, if the nature of medical data, such as survival times in ALS.MND patients taking a particular experimental treatment versus those taking placebo, precludes the use of methods that assume that such observations are normally distributed, the *means* for such a sample are distributed normally. Observations from recent Duchenne dystrophy cooperative trials are relevant to ALS.MND clinical trials, e.g., the use of ANOVA and the *F* statistic in such trials and the comparison among interval, nominal, and ordinal data. Interval data, as being explored by Munsat and colleagues in the TQNE (32), uses actual height, whereas nominal data present information as either right-handed or left-handed. Ordinal data, as used in scales, such as the MRC scales for strength and the disability scales (Norris, Appel, ALSSS, Japanese, etc.) can only provide mild, moderate, and severe analysis. Different statistical methods are required depending on whether the data are interval, nominal, or ordinal, e.g., for interval data when two different results are compared, the unpaired Student's *t* test is used, whereas Chi-square is used for nominal and Mann-Whitney rank sum is used for ordinal data, respectively. When more than two values are compared for interval data, ANOVA is used, while Chi-square and Kruskal-Wallis tests are used for nominal and ordinal observations, respectively. The types of errors possible in such trials indicate that such considerations must really be discussed at length with biostatisticians unfamiliar with ALS.MND prior to the final drafting of the treatment trial protocol. Such discussions are extremely important when a negative result in such a trial is found and the authors wish to communicate their conclusions. In such instances, it is essential to calculate the power of the study in order to accurately predict the change. Such considerations involve formulas that ascertain type *beta* and type *alpha* errors (false negatives and false positives, respectively).

Robinson (Chapter 20) has begun a preliminary evaluation of an ALS.MND database. Such databases have previously been constructed in the United States and Japan but have not been given much of an enthusiastic response. They are costly, severely limited, and labor intensive, but new consideration of modified databases in international cooperative studies may be possible. Funding for such databases might come from the World Health Organization (WHO), the World Federation of Neurology (WFN), and other groups. Along these lines, a subcommittee of the WFN Research Group on Neuromuscular Disease to deal with ALS.MND clinical trials has been formed with Dr. Munsat as its chairman. The full subcommittee is currently being formed and was announced at the WFN 12th World Congress of Neurology in Delhi, India, October 1989.

TRIAL DESIGN AND ASSESSMENT

Guiloff (Chapter 3) emphasizes aspects essential to the concepts of experimental treatment trials in ALS.MND, e.g., drugs that might be tried in these patients might be directed at the cause(s) and/or the mechanisms leading to motor neuron loss and/or the mechanisms causing the symptoms and signs displayed by patients. Furthermore, investigators should not assume that drugs would have similar actions on both normal and diseased motor neurons or muscle. It should likewise not be assumed that a drug would have similar effects on *all* motor neurons (i.e., cortical, bulbar, and spinal) or that a drug would have similar effects at all stages of the illness in a given patient or in patients with different progression rates.

Consideration must also be given to expectations by patients and investigators as to what exactly is meant by treatment. Is it to decrease mortality, and/or to increase survival time? Is it to decrease progression rate, and/or to increase symptomatic improvement? As always, it is the responsibility of the physician to first do no harm (primum non nocere).

In trial design, the options of open versus controlled need to be considered. Open trials may be acute or subacute, whereas placebo-controlled trials can be random with parallel or crossover designs. The need to have adequately matched controls for ALS.MND trials and the vagaries of assessment difficulties have been previously discussed (35).

HOPE FOR THE FUTURE

As indicated above, there is much hope for the future for ALS.MND clinical trials. This is the age of recombinant molecules in clinical trial research. This era was ushered in for ALS.MND trials by the recently completed multicenter recombinant human growth hormone (rhGH; Protropin) trial (36). A host of molecules, with relevance to the nervous system, have been cloned and produced by recombinant techniques: rNGF (nerve growth factor), rIGF-1 (insulin-like growth factor-1; somatomedin C), rPDGF (platelet-derived growth factor), and rEGF (epidermal growth factor), to list just a few. With improvement in measurement techniques such as TQNE, computer modeling, and so forth, and general improvement in ALS.MND trial design, the time required before testing such agents in patients with ALS.MND will increasingly shrink. This is reason enough to be optimistic for the future.

Acknowledgment: The author is grateful to the patients and families who recently completed the first multicenter trial of a recombinant molecule (rhGH) in ALS.MND; to Bill Parlette and the ALS.MND Research Foundation, and to colleagues R.A. Smith, S. Melmed, B. Sherman, T.L. Munsat, F.H. Norris, and F.C. Rose for their encouragement and collegiality; and to Lori Peterson, for the preparation of this manuscript. Support for the rhGH (Protropin) trial came from Genentech, Inc., and the Muscular Dystrophy Association.

REFERENCES

1. Mulder DW. *The diagnosis and treatment of amyotrophic lateral sclerosis.* Boston: Houghton Mifflin, 1980.
2. Festoff BW, Crigger NJ. Therapeutic trials in amyotrophic lateral sclerosis: a review. In: Mulder DW, ed. *The diagnosis and treatment of amyotrophic lateral sclerosis.* Boston: Houghton Mifflin, 1980:337–69.
3. Engel WK, Siddique T, Nicoloff JT. Effect on weakness and spasticity in amyotrophic lateral sclerosis of thyrotropin-releasing hormone. *Lancet* 1983;2:73–5.
4. Imoto K, Saida K, Iwamura K, et al. Amyotrophic lateral sclerosis: a double-blind crossover trial of thyrotropin-releasing hormone. *J Neurol Neurosurg Psychiatry* 1985;47:159–61.
5. Mitsumoto H, Salgado ED, Negroski D, et al. Trials of thyrotropin-releasing hormone (TRH) treatment in patients with amyotrophic lateral sclerosis. *Neurology* 1986; 36:152–9.
6. Munsat TL, Bradley WJ. In: Tyler HR, Darvison PM, eds. *Current neurology.* Boston: Houghton Mifflin, 1979:79–103.
7. Appel SH. A unifying hypothesis for the cause of amyotrophic lateral sclerosis, parkinsonism and Alzheimer's disease. *Ann Neurol* 1981;10:499–505.
8. Festoff BW. Approaches to modern therapeutic clinical trials in ALS. In: Rose FC, ed. *Research progress in motor neurone disease* London: Pitman, 1984:432–42.
9. Spencer PS, Schaumburg HH, Cohn DF, Seth PK. Lathyrism: a useful model of primary lateral sclerosis. In: Rose FC, ed. *Research progress in motor neurone disease.* London: Pitman, 1984:312–27.
10. Koerner DR. Abnormal carbohydrate metabolism in amyotrophic lateral sclerosis and parkinsonism–dementia on Guam. *Diabetes* 1976;25:1055–65.
11. Reyes ET, Perurena OH, Festoff BW, Popiela H. Role of insulin receptors and insulin insensitivity in amyotrophic lateral sclerosis and related diseases. In: Rose FC, ed. *Research progress in motor neurone disease.* London: Pitman, 1984:263–75.

12. Calne DB, McGeer E, Eisen A, Spencer P. Alzheimer's disease, Parkinson's disease, and motoneurone disease: abiotrophic interaction between ageing and environment? *Lancet* 1986;1:1067–70.
13. Perurena OH, Festoff BW. Reduction in insulin receptors in amyotrophic lateral sclerosis correlates with reduced insulin sensitivity. *Neurology* 1987;37:1375–9.
14. Spencer PS, Nunn PB, Hugon J, et al. Guam amyotrophic lateral sclerosis-parkinsonism-dementia linked to a plant excitant neurotoxin. *Science* 1987;23:517–22.
15. Spencer PS, Ludolph A, Dwivedi MP, Roy DN, Jugon J, Schaumburg HH. Lathyrism: evidence for role of the neuroexcitatory amino acid BOAA. *Lancet* 1986;1:1066–70.
16. Plaitakis A, Caroscio JT. Abnormal glutamate metabolism in amyotrophic lateral sclerosis. *Ann Neurol* 1987;22:575–9.
17. Perry TL, Hansen S, Jones K. Brain glutamate deficiency in amyotrophic lateral sclerosis. *Neurology* 1987;37:1845–8.
18. Festoff BW, Fernandez HL. Plasma and red blood cell acetylcholinesterase in amyotrophic lateral sclerosis. *Muscle Nerve* 1981;4:41–7.
19. Rasool CG, Bradley WG, Connolly B, and Baruah JK. Acetylcholinesterase and ATPase in motor neuron degenerative diseases. *Muscle Nerve* 1983;6:430–5.
20. Tandan R, Bradley WG. Amyotrophic lateral sclerosis: part 2. Etiopathogenesis. *Ann Neurol* 1985;18:419–31.
21. Rowland LP. Diverse forms of motor neuron disease. In: Rowland LP, ed. *Human motor neuron diseases*, vol 36. New York: Raven Press, 1982:1–11.
22. Rose FC (ed). *Research progress in motor neurone disease*. London: Pitman, 1984.
23. Cosi V, Kato AC, Parlette W, Pinelli P, Poloni M (eds). *Amyotrophic lateral sclerosis: therapeutic, psychological and research aspects*. New York: Plenum Press, 1987.
24. Tsubaki T, Yase Y (eds). *Amyotrophic lateral sclerosis: recent advances in research and treatment*. Amsterdam: Elsevier, 1988.
25. Aran FA. Recherches sur une maladie non encore decrite du système musculaire (atrophie musculaire progressive). *Arch Gèn Mèd* 1850;24:5–35.
26. Duchenne G. Paralysie musculaire progressive de la langue, du voile de palaise et des lèvres. *Arch Gèn Mèd* 1860;16:283,431.
27. Charcot JM, Joffroy A. Deux cas d'atrophie musculaire progressive avec lésions de la substance grise et des faiseceaux antérolatèraux de la moelle épinière. *Arch Physiol* 1869;2:354, 629, 744.
28. Appel V, Stewart SS, Smith G, Appel SH. A rating scale for amyotrophic lateral sclerosis: description and preliminary experience. *Ann Neurol* 1987;22:328–33.
29. Brooke MH, Fenichel GM, Griggs RC, et al. Clinical investigation of Duchenne muscular dystrophy. *Arch Neurol* 1987;44:812–7.
30. Feinstein AR. *Clinimetrics*. New Haven: Yale University Press, 1987.
31. Norris FH, Calanchini PR, Fallat RJ, et al. The administration of guanidine in amyotrophic lateral sclerosis. *Neurology* 1974;24:721–8.
32. Andres PL, Hedlund W, Finison LJ, Conlon T, Felnus M, Munsat TL. Quantitative motor assessment in amyotrophic lateral sclerosis. *Neurology* 1986;36:937–41.
33. Stalberg E. Recent progress in ALS neurophysiology. In: Tsubaki T, Yase Y (eds). *Amyotrophic lateral sclerosis: recent advances in research and treatment*. Amsterdam: Elsevier, 1988: 155–60.
34. Matthews DE, Farewell VT. *Using and understanding medical statistics* (2nd ed). Basel: Karger, 1988.

35. Rose FC. Clinical trials in motor neurone disease (MND). In: Tsubaki T, Yase Y, eds. *Amyotrophic lateral sclerosis: recent advances in research and treatment.* Amsterdam: Elsevier, 1988.
36. Festoff BW, Smith RA, Melmed S. Therapeutic trial of recombinant human growth hormone in amyotrophic lateral sclerosis. In: Serratrice G, ed., *Neuromuscular diseases,* 1989 (in press).

Amyotrophic Lateral Sclerosis,
edited by F. Clifford Rose.
Demos Publications, New York © 1990.

2

Nomenclature, Definition, and Classification

Sebastian Conradi

Department of Neurology, Karolinska Sjukhuset, 104 01 Stockholm, Sweden

Amyotrophic lateral sclerosis (ALS), or motor neuron disease (MND) as it is also called in some regions, kills about 10,000 persons annually in Europe and the United States, most of whom die within 3–5 years from onset. The situation of the ALS patient is indeed critical and practically unique in modern medicine, due to the poor prognosis, disabling symptoms, and a remarkable lack of curative treatment (as well as a lack of clinical trials). ALS patients have proven to be a medical enigma, and medicine's inadequacy in treating these patients because of the lack of information available about the disease has caused some physicians to avoid treating them, which in turn impedes medical care.

Although the basic cause of the disease is still unknown, knowledge regarding ALS has increased in recent years, and many theories on the pathophysiology and suggestions of treatment have been presented. Therapeutic trials in ALS are urgent, not only because they can increase knowledge of the disease, but also because trials often improve the medical care of participating patients. Trials of treatment during the early stages of the disease offer several advantages: many new symptoms appear during treatment, and these can be evaluated. The period of observation can be extended, and this is advantageous, since symptom progress represents a very indirect measure of the pathophysiological process and there could be a delay between onset of treatment and clinical effect. Criteria are required for diagnosis and classification that can be applied in early cases, and not include the progression of the disease to its final stages.

NOMENCLATURE

Unfortunately, the nomenclature of ALS or MND is a subject of controversy and confusion. The disease is called ALS in most countries, but the term MND is preferred in Great Britain. It is important to agree on one name for this disease to avoid further confusion.

The term MND has several disadvantages as follows.

It is inexact. There is not just one but several motor neuron diseases. Further, the disease does not affect all motor neurons, since gamma - and preganglionic autonomic motor neurons are mildly-affected if at all (1). It has also been shown in recent years that the disease may involve not only motor neurons but also other types of neurons, for example large sensory neurons (2) and neurons in Clarke's column (3).

It is a mixture of Latin and English. The term includes "disease," which is English, although "motor neuron" is Latin. Neutrality of language is preferred, and the construction of this term also causes difficulties in abbreviations in other languages.

ALS, the name used most frequently, also has several disadvantages.

It is difficult to understand. The full Latin name is long and is difficult to pronounce and understand. Further, the name may sound mysterious and probably threatening to most patients. It is preferably used in the abbreviated form, as are several other diseases known to the public, e.g., MS and AIDS.

It is incorrect. The name ALS is incorrect in the most commonly used meaning, i.e., a disease of motor neurons that has at least three clinical subtypes. One type affects both central and peripheral motor neurons (ALS), a second subtype predominantly affects bulbar motor neurons [bulbar paralysis (BP)] and in a third subtype, just peripheral spinal motor neurons [progressive spinal muscle atrophy (PMA)] are involved. In PMA, there is, by definition, no symptoms caused by sclerosis of the lateral columns of the spinal cord, as the term ALS implies.

It has a double meaning. The most serious disadvantage of the name ALS is that it has a double meaning, since it is both a general term for the disease and for one of the clinical subtypes. This fact causes much confusion not only in the scientific literature but also in medical education and in informing patients. The term ALS proper (ALSp) or classic ALS can be used for the clinical subtype that has symptoms from peripheral spinal and central spinal and bulbar motor neurons, and in some cases also symptoms from peripheral bulbar motor neurons. The major problems with ALS are its etiology and finding an effective treatment, which should not be obscured by discussions on nomenclature. The term ALS is used most frequently, and it is suggested that this term should receive general acceptance, provided the problem with the nomenclature of the subtypes can be solved.

DEFINITION

The characteristic symptoms of ALS are easy for the trained neurologist to recognize (4), especially when the patient has suffered from the disease for some time; these symptoms will not be discussed in detail here. Sometimes there are difficulties in early cases but, as has been mentioned, there are several reasons for including early cases of ALS in therapeutic trials. Due to improved medical standards in recent years, many patients will attend a neurologic specialist early in the disease course, and we have seen many cases within a few months from onset of weakness showing symptoms from just one or a few muscles.

Symptoms and Signs

In most cases, the diagnosis will rely on a triad of factors: (a) presence of progressive neuromuscular symptoms and signs, (b) results of investigations with electromyography (EMG) and electroneurography (ENeG), and (c) exclusion of other diseases. Of these three, the nature of symptoms and signs is least controversial, since they can practically always be described with one or several of the terms: weakness, atrophy, spasticity, fasciculations, and cramps.

EMG and ENeG Studies

The EMG changes found in clinically unaffected muscles are especially important in early cases. There seems to be no generally accepted formal criteria for the nature and spread of the changes required to confirm the diagnosis of ALS.

The character of neurogenic changes (large motor unit potentials of irregular shape, loss of motor units, fibrillation potentials and, in ALS, often also fasciculations) seems to arouse no controversy between investigators. The most important question for the clinician is the number and location of the muscles studied and how much acute denervation (fibrillation) is required. Several workers in the field (such as our own group) demand EMG recordings from both proximal and distal muscles in all four extremities but not from the abdomen or head and neck. So far, we have required neurogenic changes not being restricted to distal muscles (to rule out polyneuropathy) from three extremities in nonbulbar patients to accept the ALS diagnosis. In BP patients, neurogenic changes from two recording sites are often sufficient because bulbar paresis is such a characteristic symptom. These requirements have fulfilled a practical purpose and work well. On occasion it is necessary to wait for more generalized changes, and occasional BP patients have initially shown no neurogenic changes or occurrence of acute denervation (fibrillations) in the extremities. Fasciculations seem to vary to a great extent between patients;

it might be difficult to include any requirement of them to accept the diagnosis. It is important that the EMG and ENeG (discussed below) criteria for early ALS diagnosis are discussed further so that international agreement can be reached.

Conventionally, the motor and sensory conduction velocities on ENeG are described to be normal in ALS or to show some distal reduction of motor nerve conduction velocity due to sprouting (5). The clinician meets with difficulties in such cases where there are disseminated neurogenic EMG findings as in ALS plus reduced conduction velocity in motor (and sometimes sensory) nerves. Due to the uncertainty of the character of such cases (discussed below) it might be advantageous to exclude them from clinical trials.

Differential Diagnosis

During periods of the disease, especially in early stages, ALS may resemble some other diseases, and early diagnosis will sometimes require exclusion of these conditions. However, it might be difficult to standardize completely the tests required. The conditions that most frequently cause diagnostic problems are: (a) Charcot-Marie-Tooth disease (CMT), (b) some forms of polyneuropathy including chronic Guillain-Barré syndrome, (c) spondyloarthrosis, especially in the cervical region, (d) Lyme disease, and (e) myositis and syringobulbia.

The differentiation between early ALS and Type 1 CMT cases rests on the presence in ALS of neurogenic EMG findings proximally in the extremities and no or only slight changes on neurography. Differentiation toward Type 2 CMT will rely on EMG findings only but the clinical distinction between the two conditions is not always absolute. Differentiation especially between PMA and chronic Guillain-Barré syndrome requires neurography and cerebrospinal fluid (CSF) analysis, which otherwise have limited value in diagnosing ALS. There are earlier descriptions of raised CSF total protein in ALS (6), which can make this differentiation difficult. Spondyloarthrosis, besides giving a clinical picture that is very similar to ALS, may also induce changes in the clinical course of the disease, e.g., by adding symptoms from the pyramidal tract to PMA cases, thereby giving a false subtype. Cervical myelography may be needed in such cases, although this investigation cannot be required generally.

There is a great need for a chemical laboratory test to improve early diagnosis in ALS. A cytotoxic activity in the plasma of ALS patients which induces an increased hemolysis in normal erythrocytes has been described in our laboratory (7). The activity that persists in isolated immunoglobulins (Ig) of ALS patients and can be characterized further in a series of plasma dilutions (8) has now been demonstrated to occur in greater than 95% of approximately 250 consecutive cases of ALS in an early stage of the disease. This activity is not found in plasma of normal controls (approximately 150 cases) and neurological controls (CMT, Guillain-Barré syndrome, traumatic paraplegia) but can be found in cases of

Kugelberg-Welander's spinal muscle atrophy (unpublished observations). Laboratory tests for ALS will in the future answer the question of whether the pathogenetic process in ALS can also induce disease states outside the clinical limitations of ALS as seen today. Examples of such diseases are cases with ALS-like symptoms in just a few muscles (9), reversible ALS-like cases (10), ALS-like symptoms under the age of 20, and patients with symptoms and EMG findings of ALS, but showing reduced motor (and sensory) conduction velocities together with conduction blocks (11). Cases such as these have shown cytotoxic activity directed toward erythrocytes in our laboratory. Although of great theoretical interest, such patients cannot at present be used in therapeutic trials in ALS.

CLASSIFICATION

From a global perspective, ALS has three forms: sporadic, hereditary, and Western Pacific (Guam) ALS. Our interest centers on first-hand sporadic and hereditary cases, which can obviously be included in therapeutic studies. Division of ALS into clinical subtypes has two main implications: (a) the subtypes have a different prognosis, (b) the difference in symptoms between the subtypes indicates that the pathophysiological process has at least three modes of operation (discussed below). In addition to clinical subtype, only age and initial rate of symptom progression appear to be predictive in prognosis (12,13): an early classification of ALS patients into clinical subtype is therefore important in the evaluation of therapy. As mentioned, there are conventionally three main clinical subtypes: BP, ALSp, and PMA. In most texts, primary lateral sclerosis (PLS) is described as a fourth subtype, but, since these cases are uncommon, diagnosis is difficult, and early diagnosis cannot rely on EMG findings, these cases have limited practical interest in therapeutic studies.

One semantic difficulty involves the use of BP in early subtype classification of ALS patients. BP is interchangeably used as a symptom and as a notation of a clinical subtype. As a symptom BP can be a rather late manifestation in cases starting with peripheral and central spinal symptoms (i.e. ALSp). In some series, these cases are dealt with separately. This confusion is probably one reason why the proportion of BP cases varies considerably between different series of ALS patients. Since a clinical classification for treatment purposes has to rely on early symptoms, it seems reasonable to reserve the term BP for that subtype of ALS in which bulbar symptoms present early in the disease.

Unfortunately, the term BP is connected with yet another semantic problem. In cases with early bulbar symptoms (BP subtype), it is not clear whether the spinal symptoms of this subtype should be both central and peripheral or whether cases with only peripheral spinal symptoms should also be included. In our experience, the few cases with only peripheral, bulbospinal symptoms

Table 2-1. *Symptoms in Clinical Subtypes of ALS*

	Peripheral		Central	
Clinical subtype	Bulbar	Spinal	Bulbar	Spinal
PMA	–	2+	–	–
ALSp	+/–	2+	+	2+
BP	2+	+	2+/(–)	+/(–)
PLS	–	(+)	2+	2+

(bulbospinal muscle atrophy) often have a much more benign course than most other BP cases.

The classification of ALS cases into clinical subtypes is based on the occurrence and time course of symptoms from peripheral spinal and bulbar neurons and central spinal and bulbar neurons, respectively (Table 2-1). As seen in Table 2-1, the different modes of action of the pathogenetic process in ALS can in all probability operate independently. It might well be that treatment regimens will interact in different ways on the various kinds of symptoms (e.g., that peripheral spinal symptoms are more easily accessible to treatment than other symptoms). This, in turn, makes it highly desirable to develop scoring methods that evaluate the symptoms from the three neuronal systems separately.

In conclusion, there is a great need for generally accepted criteria regarding nomenclature, definition, and classification that can be applied especially in early ALS cases. Such criteria will help improve therapeutic trials.

REFERENCES

1. Sobue K, Matsuoka Y, Mukai E, Takayanagi T, Sobue I, Hashizume Y. Spinal and cranial motor nerve roots in amyotrophic lateral sclerosis and x-linked recessive bulbospinal muscular atrophy. Morphometric and teased-fiber study. *Acta Neuropathol (Berl)* 1981;55:227–35.
2. Dyck PJ, Stevens JC, Mulder DW, Espinosa RE. Frequency of nerve fiber degeneration of peripheral motor and sensory neurons in amyotrophic lateral sclerosis. *Neurology* 1975;25:781–85.
3. Averback P, Crocker P. Regular involvement of Clarke's nucleus in sporadic amyotrophic lateral sclerosis. *Arch Neurol* 1982;39:155–56.
4. Rowland LP. Diverse forms of motor neuron diseases. In: Rowland LP, ed. Human motor neuron diseases. New York: Raven Press, 1982:1–11 (Advances in neurology; vol 36.).
5. Lambert EH. Electromyography in amyotrophic lateral sclerosis. In: Norris FH, Kurland LT, eds. *Motor neuron diseases.* New York: Grune & Stratton, 1969:135–53.

6. Guiloff RJ, McGregor B, Thompson E, Blackwood W, Paul E. Motor neuron disease with elevated cerebrospinal fluid protein. *J Neurol Neurosurg Psychiatry* 1980;43:390–96.
7. Conradi S, Ronnevi L-O. Cytotoxic activity in the plasma of amyotrophic lateral sclerosis (ALS) patients against normal erythrocytes. Quantitative determination *J Neurol Sci* 1985;68:135–45.
8. Ronnevi L-O, Conradi S, Karlsson E, Sindhupak R. Nature and properties of cytotoxic plasma activity in amyotrophic lateral sclerosis. *Muscle Nerve* 1987;10:734–43.
9. Compernolle T. A case of juvenile muscular atrophy confined to one upper limb. *Eur Neurol* 1973;10:237–42.
10. Mitchell DM, Olczak SA. Remission of a syndrome indistinguishable from motor neuron disease after resection of bronchial carcinoma. *Br Med J* 1979;2:176–77.
11. Lewis RA, Sumner AJ, Brown MJ, Asbury AK. Multifocal demyelinating neuropathy with persistent conduction block. *Neurology* 1982;32:958–64.
12. Cariosco JT, Calhoun WF, Yahr MD. Prognostic factors in motor neuron disease: a prospective study of longevity. In: Rose FC, ed. *Research progress in motor neuron disease.* London: Pitman, 1984:34–43.
13. Munsat TL, Andres PL, Finison L, Conlon T, Thibodeau L. The natural history of motor neuron loss in amyotrophic lateral sclerosis. *Neurology* 1988;38:409–13.

Amyotrophic Lateral Sclerosis,
edited by F. Clifford Rose.
Demos Publications, New York © 1990.

Motor Neuron Disease: Aims and Assessment Methods in Trial Design

R.J. Guiloff, H. Modarres-Sadeghi, and H. Rogers

Department of Neurology, Westminster Hospital, Charing Cross and Westminster Medical School, London, England

Ideally, clinical workers in motor neuron disease (MND) would like to find a drug that, like penicillin for pneumococcal pneumonia, would arrest disease progression and restore anatomy and neurological function by its action on the cause of the disease. Presently there is no clue as to the cause of the disease, and neurons and neurological function cannot be restored once lost. Attempts to treat MND may follow a number of leads but the answers are heavily dependent on the questions asked and the methods chosen to answer them.

There are many examples of (currently) incurable diseases for which a variety of strategies have resulted in significant advances in management. Levodopa treatment for Parkinson's disease results in prolonged symptomatic improvement, and age-related mortality has been reduced nearly threefold since the prelevodopa era, to almost equal that of the general population. Cholinergic agents, steroids, and other immunosuppressants, plasmapheresis, and thymectomy may all play a role in the symptomatic treatment of myasthenia gravis. Survival in many cancers and in certain leukemias has been significantly increased by the use of chemotherapy, radiotherapy, or bone marrow transplants.

Short of finding a complete cure for MND (as defined above), the design of drug trials and the assessment methods used need to be tailored to the treatment aims pursued with a particular agent. This requires explicit statements about what is perceived or meant by treatment in MND.

Provided it does not produce serious side-effects, a given drug may be useful in MND for a variety of reasons: (a) it may produce prolonged symptomatic improvements, (b) it may reduce the rate of deterioration in one or more affected functions, (c) it may prolong survival time, and (d) it may reduce the mortality rate of the disease. One or more of these possible beneficial effects might be due to an action of the drug on the cause of the disease, on the mechanisms leading to motor neuron loss or dysfunction, or on the mechanisms mediating symptom production related to such motor neuron loss or dysfunction. Drugs might exert these actions, directly or indirectly, on cortical, bulbar, or spinal motor neurons and/or their connections (1).

There is no *a priori* reason why a given drug should have similar actions on cortical, bulbar, or spinal motor neurons, or in cervical and lumbar enlargement motor neurons, or in all bulbar motor cranial nerve nuclei. Even the location and synaptic connectivity of the motor neurons that innervate proximal and distal muscles in a limb are different (2). A good example of differential actions of a drug in one anatomical structure is anticholinesterase agents in myasthenia gravis. These agents may be effective only in the neuromuscular junction of certain muscles, whereas function may deteriorate in others at the same time. Theoretically, a drug effect on any one of the four beneficial actions mentioned above may, or may not, be associated with effects in one or more of the others. For example, an agent might have an effect on limb motor neuron function with significant improvement in somatic disability; survival time and mortality, which are closely related to respiratory and bulbar function, would remain unchanged (3). Another might have a symptomatic action on bulbar and high cervical cord motor neuron function; if this effect is prolonged, survival time may be longer, although somatic disability and mortality would be unchanged. Yet another might reduce the rate of deterioration in bulbar and respiratory function without any detectable symptomatic improvement or effect on mortality but with prolongation of survival time. (The reader may think of other possible situations.) Unless the clinical researcher takes into account these considerations when planning the design and assessment methods used in a trial with a new agent, it may be difficult to decide later in what respect that drug was, or was not, useful.

ASSESSMENT METHODS

Whatever the trial design, the value of the information analyzed will depend on the assessment methods used. The detailed discussion on the sensibility of a clinical index for MND that includes its purpose and framework, comprehensibility, replicability, suitability of the scale used, face validity, content validity, and ease of usage (4) is beyond the scope of this chapter. Whichever scales are used, they should allow for adequate separate assessments of bulbar, high cervical, and upper and lower limb function. For the reasons stated earlier, and depending on the weight given to the various items, a global scale may indicate deterioration when it is occurring, for example, only in limb function and a potential drug is having a significant effect on bulbar or high cervical cord functions.

Of all assessment methods, probably the most important ones are those

Table 3-1. *Clinical Features of Patients*

Patient/ age/sex	Form	Norris Scale	Tinc	Dur	Main Disability	Bulbar: Speech	Bulbar: Tongue	Bulbar: Jaw	Bulbar: Swal	VC: Mean ± S)	Weakness: UL	Weakness: LL	Spasticity: UL	Spasticity: LL
1/47/M	ALS	84		38	Hand weakness	1	S_2LM_1	S_2	1	2.5 ± 0.3	3	0	0	0
2/69/F	B	84	14	17	Dysarthria	3	S_3LM_1	S_2LM_1	2	1.3 ± 0.2	2	1	0	0
3/45/M	B	70	8	14	Dysarthria	3	S_3LM_1	S_2	3	3.3 ± 0.3	3	1	0	0
4/63/M	B	92		13	Dysarthria	2	S_2LM_1	S_1	1	2.7 ± 0.3	1	0	0	0
5/34/M	ALS	55	25	32	Arm weakness	1	S_2LM_1	S_1	1	2.4 ± 0.4	3	0	1	3
6/53/M	ALS	86		28	Dysarthria	1	S_1	S_1	1	4.3 ± 0.4	1	0	1	2
7/56/F	B	93		18	Dysarthria	2	S_2LM_1	S_1	1	1.4 ± 0.4	1	1	0	0
8/48/M	ALS	78	24	96	Arm weakness	1	S_1LM_2	S_1	1	3.3 ± 0.4	3	0	0	0
9/32/F	ALS	34	48	72	Tetraplegia	2	S_1	S_2	2	0.8 ± 0.3	3	3	3	0
10/58/M	ALS	75		7	Hand weakness	1	S_1LM_1	S_1	1	2.5 ± 0.2	2	1	0	0

TINC, time to severe incapacity (months): DUR, duration of illness (months); SWAL, swallowing; VC, vital capactiy (l); ALS, amyotrophic lateral sclerosis, B, bulbar; S, spasticity; LM, lower motor neuron features; UL, upper limb; LL, lower limb: Impairment grading: 0, nil; 1, mild; 2, moderate; 3, severe.

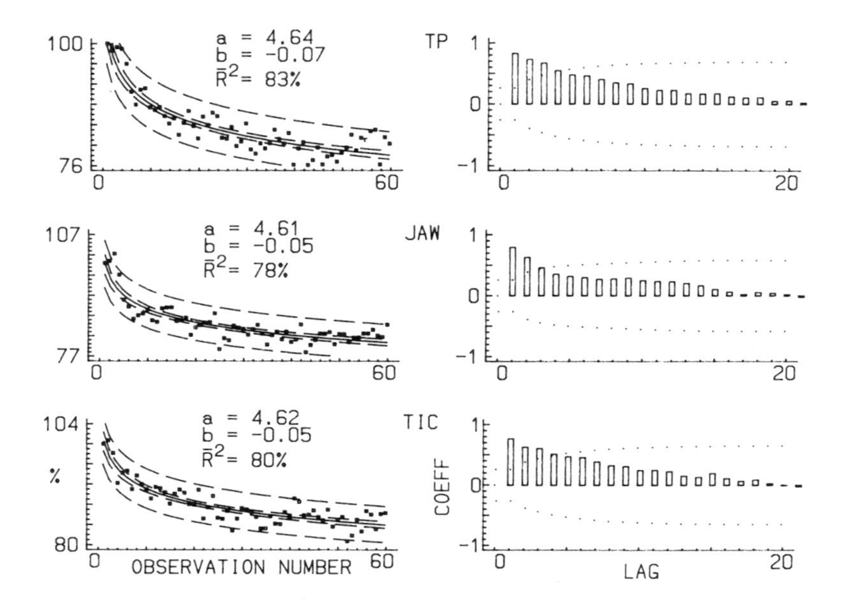

FIG. 3-1. *Bulbar function baselines. Learning effects in 10 MND patients.* Timed measurements of tongue protrusion (TP), jaw opening (JAW), and repetition of the word "ticker" (TIC) were made. There were 20 assessments of each function with 3 replications at each assessment point, over 7–10 days. A total of 60 observations were thus made for each function. The data for each patient were expressed as a percentage of the first observation. At each observation point in the time series, the mean percentage for the 10 patients has been plotted. **Left column:** The central (solid) line is fitted for a multiplicative model ($y = ax^b$) with its 95% confidence limits and those of the means at each observation point (broken lines). Percentages below 100 indicate less time to perform the test than on the first observation (i.e. learning). Obvious learning occurs until about observation No. 30. **Right column:** The autocorrelation functions for the same data are shown. Dotted lines represent the boundaries below which the autocorrelation coefficients (bars) at each lag are not significantly different from 0. The initial three or four coefficients are outside these limits for the time series of 60 observations. This situation persists when the autocorrelation is repeated, sequentially dropping values from the beginning of the series, until observation 27–30 is used as the starting point for the analysis i.e., learning effect no longer present (not shown).

measuring bulbar and high cervical cord function. Although somatic involvement in MND (trunk and limbs) becomes disabling, survival time and mortality will relate closely to the advent of respiratory failure and to impairment of bulbar functions such as swallowing. We shall consider here some aspects of the clinical assessment of bulbar function that are relevant to drug trials. Some

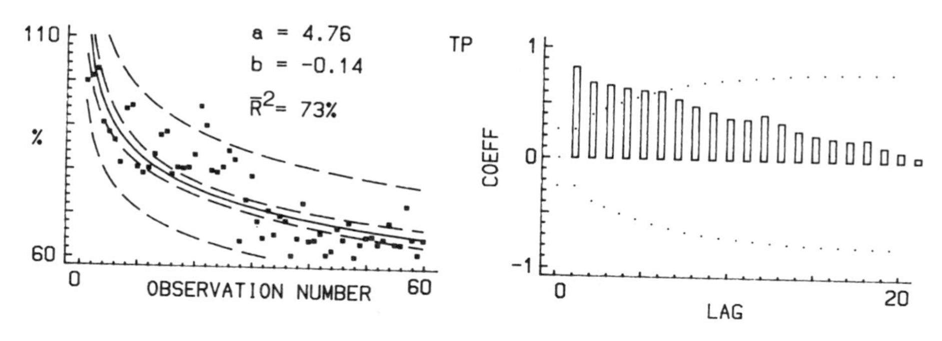

FIG. 3-2. *Baseline for tongue protrusion in patient 1. Learning effects.* See legend to Fig. 3-1 for details.

of the problems relating to the assessment of limb function, in particular measurements of muscle force have been discussed recently (5) and elsewhere in this volume.

Common to all assessment methods is the need to have reliable baselines. Changes in function should be measured in relation to them. For some timed measurements of bulbar function, significant learning effects are present in the baselines and should be eliminated before comparisons with measurements after drug and placebo administration are made. Table 3-1 lists the main features of 10 patients with MND with bulbar syndrome. Figure 3-1 shows learning effects in their baselines when measuring timed tongue protrusion, jaw opening, and word repetition using a multiplicative model and an autocorrelation function. A similar analysis for one function tested in one of the patients is shown in Fig. 3-2. By using quality control techniques such as the cumulative sum procedure (6), it is possible to study a completed time series, as the one containing baseline assessments, and judge the presence of significant learning effects, that is, values that are outside defined control limits. By individual elimination of a variable number of initial measurements, the shortened baselines may be shown to contain no values outside the defined limits, either with the combined data of the 10 patients or in an individual case (Fig. 3-3). In a drug trial situation, it may be necessary to look at the time series as it unfolds, defining the critical bounds from the standard deviation of the mean baseline values and using a recursive coefficient to establish the presence, or absence, of learning effects during baseline measurements (1,7) (Fig. 3-4).

A number of parameters may not show such learning effects. Baselines for respiratory parameters and timed swallowing are good examples and are shown for the same 10 patients in Fig. 3-5.

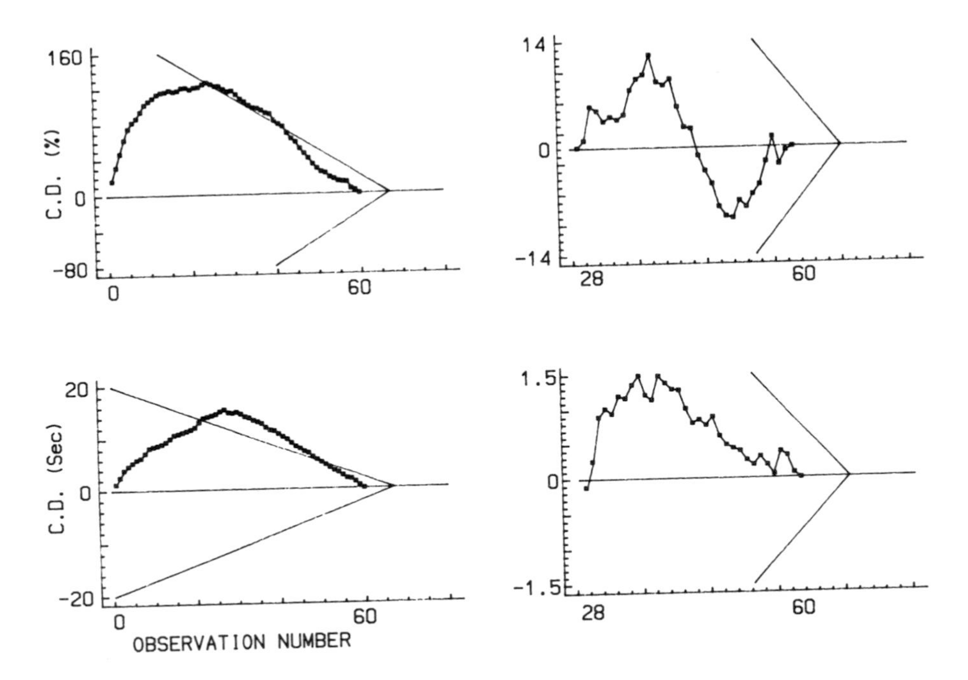

FIG. 3-3. *Cumulative sum plots. Baselines for tongue protrusion in 10 MND patients. Learning effect.* **Top row:** On the *left,* mean values for 10 patients normalized as a percentage of the first observation in each individual were used. The cumulative sum of the difference from the mean of the completed time series is plotted at each observation point. The V-shaped lines indicate critical bounds at 5% significance for 1 SD from mean baseline. Significant learning is shown by structural breaks in the time series between observations 20 and 40. On the *right,* when only the last 33 observations are taken, no points are outside critical bounds. **Bottom row:** Same analysis for patient 1 using this individual's measurements (untransformed data in seconds). *Left:* taking all 60 observations. *Right:* taking the last 33 observations.

The above discussion emphasizes the need to carefully define the behavior of each parameter intended for use in drug trials. This should apply to each item included in a global scale, whether ordinal or consisting of dimensional data. The more items included, the more work is needed before the scale can be reliably used. The fewer items included, the greater the chance that the scale will not be sensitive enough.

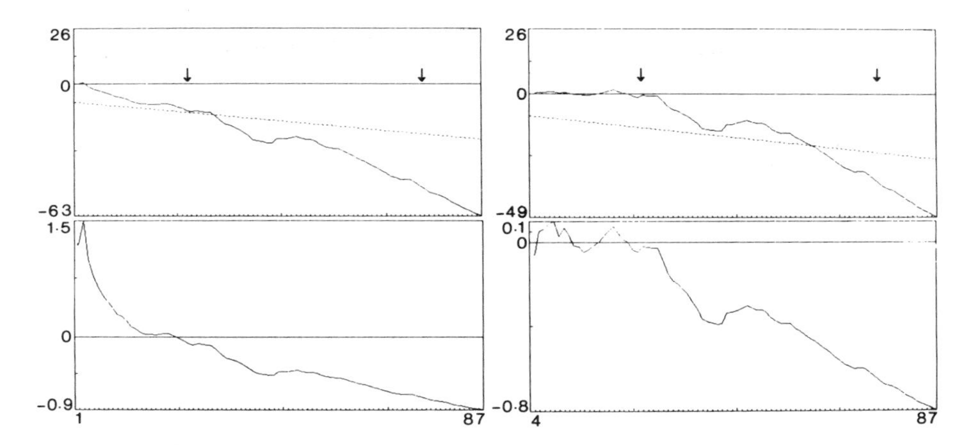

FIG. 3-4. *Learning effect. Cumulative sum. Tongue protrusion.* This case participated in a therapeutic trial (patient 3, ref.1). Left column: All data. **Right column:** After removing learning effects from the baseline. **Upper graphs:** Y axis is the cumulative sum of residuals (in seconds) with respect to mean baseline, shown for the whole time series. X axis is the serial observation number in the time series. The first and last infusions of a TRH analogue (RX77368) are indicated by arrows. Baseline period, 10 days. Post-infusion period, 7 days. The V-shaped lines indicate critical bounds at 5% significance level for 1 SD from mean baseline. **Lower graphs:** The Y axis plots the difference of each value from the mean of the process to that point. The upper left graph shows a significant structural break in the time series by point 25, that is, the cumulative sum falls below critical bounds suggesting improvement (less time to perform the test). However, the lower left graph shows a steady decline in the mean of the process during baseline indicating a learning effect. The right upper plot shows that when the first 3 of the 24 baseline values are removed the baseline is steady and there is still a significant structural break during the infusion period. The difference of each value from the mean of the process to that point now fluctuates around 0 during baseline (right lower graph).

TRIAL DESIGN

Discussions on some topics related to therapeutic trials in MND are already available, such as quality of measurements, sample size, selection of patients, randomized crossover and parallel designs, as well as ethical issues (8–10), but many issues depend on the possible aims of the drug trial in MND.

Investigation of Symptomatic Effects

Here, preliminary clinical assessments of effectiveness and toxicity in pilot open studies seem essential. The researcher will want to find out the approximate dose range required and to establish the existence of any observable beneficial acute effects. Controlled studies may follow to establish that the actions seen are not caused by placebo effects, with appropriate blinding to

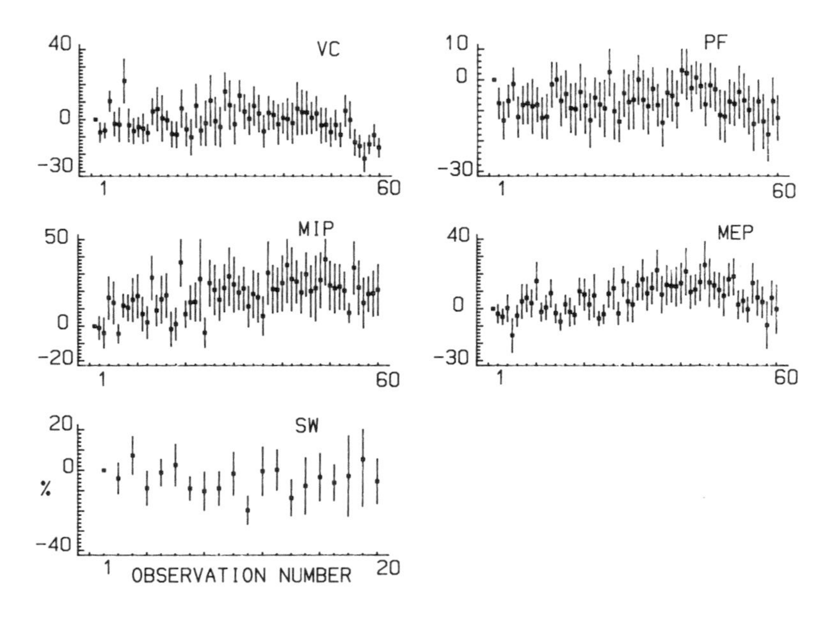

FIG. 3-5. *Baselines for respiration parameters and swallowing. Lack of learning effect in 10 MND patients.* Measurements of vital capacity (VC), peak flow (PF), and maximal inspiratory (MIP) and expiratory (MEP) pressure are described elsewhere (1). Baselines were taken as those in Fig. 3-1. For swallowing (SW), time to swallow 100 ml of water was measured once at each of 20 assessments over 7–10 days. Values are expressed as a percentage of the first observation. The points represent the mean percentage of the 10 patients and the bars 1 SE above and below that mean at each observation point.

ensure that there is no observer bias. A crossover design is preferable in these acute studies, since the number of patients required is less and it avoids the problems of matching (discussed below). Once it has been established that the desired effects are different from those of a placebo, further open trials may be necessary to find out whether the actions can be maintained and to establish the optimum dose and dose interval. Only at this stage will it be profitable to revert to a controlled design to decide whether long-term therapy (several months) with such a drug is useful; entering this phase without knowing from open medium-term studies what the optimum dose and dose interval are may lead to negative results or side-effects related to the technique of administration (e.g., cholinergic drugs in myasthenia gravis).

TABLE 3-2. *Example of Variability in Presentation and Evolution in Three Patients with MND*

Function	Patients A	Patients B	Patients C
Bulbar	Mild dysarthria	Severe dysarthria, dysphagia, and dysphonia	Normal
High cervical	Normal	Dyspnea; reduced vital capacity	Normal
Upper limbs	Weak hands	Mild proximal weakness and wasting	Normal
Lower limbs	Mild spasticity	Mild proximal weakness and wasting	Spastic paraplegia; wasting
Time from onset	2 years	9 months	5 years
Incapacity	Working	Severe exercise limitation	Wheelchair bound

The features are those at presentation in three patients seen by the authors.

Investigation of Reduction in Rate of Deterioration

It is unlikely that global scales will be sensitive and transparent enough to assess a possible action of this nature. Ordinal scales, or preferably dimensional data, which cater separately for bulbar, higher cervical cord, and upper and lower limb function are essential. The design chosen must be able to deal with clinical courses that span a 6- or 8- month to over 10-year period from clinical onset to death. Open pilot studies are required for toxicity evaluations and, in addition, may be of some help if (a) subjects with rapidly advancing disease are chosen and (b) the drug has a dramatic effect on the rate of progression of certain parameters. When an effect on rate of deterioration is not dramatic, clinical benefit may be trivial in rapidly advancing disease but worthwhile for patients with a prolonged illness. For example, a 50% reduction in rate of deterioration of respiratory function may prolong life by 4.5 months if the total clinical duration of illness would have been, say, 10 months and treatment was started in the first month. However, for somebody who started treatment after 1 year of a hypothetical illness lasting 7 years, survival would be prolonged by 3 years. The same arguments apply to other functions, like progression to severe somatic disability. Controlled trials to monitor the rate of deterioration of the above-mentioned functions over a reasonable period of time (e.g., 1 year) are therefore required.

In randomized parallel designs, matching of control (placebo) and drug groups represents a formidable problem. The variability in individual clinical

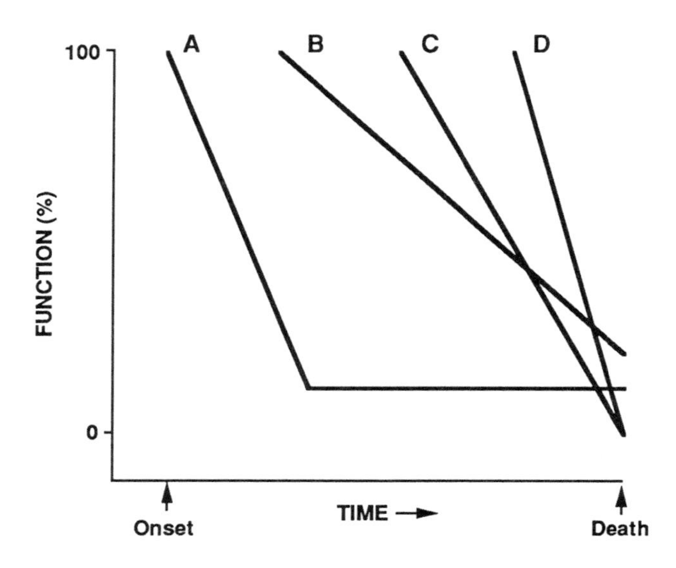

FIG. 3-6. *Variability in evolution in MND.* The graph may represent the clinical evolution of one patient with MND. Lower limb function (A) is lost rapidly, upper limb function (B) is affected later at a slower rate, a bulbar function like swallowing is affected next (C), and finally vital capacity (D) falls rapidly and the patient dies. The same graph may also exemplify the time course of deterioration in one function (e.g., lower limb) in four patients (A–D). Deterioration, when it occurs, is assumed to be linear. The time from clinical onset to death may vary from less than 1 year to over 10 years.

pictures at presentation and in patterns and time course of disease progression needs to be considered (Table 3-2). At the time of initiation of a trial, the previous evolution of the disease may have to be assumed to be linear (11,12) for each function and the time course of subsequent progression is uncertain. Clinicians are aware that in some cases the condition appears to plateau for a variable period for a certain function and that there may be no clinical involvement of other parameters also for variable amounts of time. Variability in evolution, both in the time course of a function across patients and in the pattern of functions affected in each patient, may result in a sizable number of hypothetical evolution curves being unsuitable for analysis of drug effects, since they may just produce "noise" (Fig. 3-6). This noise may represent false-positive or false-negative drug effects or lack of positive or negative effects in certain subgroups (because they are lost when analyzed together with irrelevant data for that function). A real drug effect, which could be clearly detected if linear curves of deterioration were present for each function tested and if the pattern of involvement of different functions over time was the same for all patients, will then be obscured. It may, then, be necessary to allow for eliminating a number of curves-patients so that the analysis concentrates only on those that can provide the desired information. Blind application of refined statistical methods to data that contain excessive noise may lead to lack of recognition of a true drug effect. Ethically, it may be unacceptable to have a control group and, if no benefit is apparent to the patient, large numbers of them may abandon follow up in control and drug groups.

Using a randomized crossover design avoids the problem of matching presenting clinical features and all patients receive the trial drug. It does not solve the problem of individual time course and pattern of deterioration for various functions as stated above. It is not certain even if the deterioration curves are similar for all functions in each patient, that is, if the rate of progression of the disease is the same for all motor neuronal groups in different territories.

The difficulties mentioned here may not be insoluble but will require careful attention to assessment methods, solid information about natural history and, perhaps, methods that can restrict the analysis to relevant data and eliminate noise.

Investigation of Prolongation of Survival Time

The problems of matching placebo and drug groups, in particular for bulbar and respiratory involvement at presentation and its previous rate of deterioration, will recur here since only parallel designs are adequate for this aim. Ethical considerations may be a difficulty too and, unless historical controls with careful natural history documentation exist so that matching becomes possible, it may be impossible to implement such studies.

The time of initiation of the trial can be taken as a starting point for measuring survival time. Matching must consider duration of illness, type of functions affected, and their rate of progression prior to the start point, as well as features and severity of the illness at the start point. One approach would be to follow all patients until they die. Unless only patients with rapidly evolving disease are taken, this approach would be impractical. Another approach would be to establish a fixed end point, say after 3 or 5 years and look at the median survival time of those who have died, for the samples with placebo and drug, until that end point. Assuming that progression to death relates to progression and severity of bulbar function and respiratory involvement, this progression could be measured and estimates of survival time made in the remainder.

Investigation of Reduction in Mortality Rate

A representative randomized parallel sample of patients on drug and placebo needs to be implemented and followed up. Mortality at specified periods, say 3 and 5 years, may then be compared. The problems of matching the groups and ethical difficulties will also exist here as discussed for investigation of survival time.

CONCLUSIONS

Short of finding a complete cure for motor neuron disease, clinicians need to rely on a combination of uncontrolled and controlled trials to evaluate the effects of a potential therapeutic agent. Assessment methods should be sensitive enough to answer the questions asked and to reflect the variability in clinical presentations and in patterns of evolution of bulbar, higher cervical cord, and upper and lower limb function. The importance of learning effects and of reliable baseline assessments of bulbar function are discussed. For each potential drug, prolonged symptomatic effects, prolongation of survival time, and reductions in the rate of deterioration or in mortality rate may be studied. An action in one of these items may or may not result in change in one or more of the others. Clinical trials should be tailored to study one or more of these four possible drug actions.

Acknowledgment: We are grateful to J. Emami for statistical advice and to the Motor Neurone Disease Association of Great Britain, the North West Thames Regional Health Authority, and the Special Trustees of Westminster and Roehampton Hospitals for financial support.

REFERENCES

1. Modarres-Sadeghi H, Rogers H, Emami J, Guiloff RJ. Subacute administration of a TRH analogue (RX77368) in motorneuron disease. An open study. *J Neurol Neurosurg Psychiatry* 1988;51:1146–57.
2. Kuypers HGJM. The anatomical organization of the descending pathways and their contributions to motor control especially in primates. In: Desmedt J, ed. *New developments in electromyography and clinical neurophysiology, vol 3.* Basel: Karger, 1983;36–38.
3. Guiloff RJ. TRH and motorneurone disease. *Rev Neurosci* 1987;1:201–19.
4. Feinstein AR. *Clinimetrics.* New Haven: Yale University Press, 1987.
5. Guiloff RJ, Eckland DJA. Observations on the clinical assessment of patients with motorneuron disease. Experience with a TRH analogue. *Neurol Clin* 1987;5:171–92.
6. Box GEP, Jenkins GM. *Time Series Analysis, Forecasting and Control.* San Francisco: Holden-Day, 1976.
7. Brown RL, Durbin J, Evans JM. Techniques for testing the constancy of regression relationships over time (with discussion). *J R Statistical Soc (B)* 1975;37:149–92.

8. Schoenberg BS. Controlled therapeutic trials in motor neuron disease: methodological considerations. In: Rowland LP, ed. *Human motor neuron diseases.* New York: Raven Press, 1982:547–53. (Advances in neurology; vol 36.)
9. Olarte MR. Therapeutic trials in amyotrophic lateral sclerosis. In: Rowland LP, ed. *Human motor neuron diseases.* New York: Raven Press, 1982:555–57. (Advances in neurology; vol 36.)
10. Shafer SQ, Olarte MR. Methodological considerations for clinical trials in motor neuron disease. In: Rowland LP, ed. *Human motor neuron diseases.* New York: Raven Press, 1982:559–68. (Advances in neurology; vol 36.)
11. Plaitakis A, Mandeli J, Smith J, Yahr MD. Branched-chain aminoacids in amyotrophic lateral sclerosis. *Lancet* 1988;2:680–81.
12. Guiloff RJ, Emami J. Branched-chain aminoacids in amyotrophic lateral sclerosis. *Lancet* 1988;2:680.

Amyotrophic Lateral Sclerosis,
edited by F. Clifford Rose.
Demos Publications, New York © 1990.

4

Selection of Patients in Therapeutic Trials

Mark R. Glasberg

Department of Neurology, Henry Ford Hospital, Detroit, MI, U.S.A.

Patient selection and the ability of patients to complete clinical trials are critical aspects in the success of therapeutic trials in amyotrophic lateral sclerosis (ALS). In reviewing published reports of clinical trials in ALS, there is a marked variability in the following criteria: (a) type of motor neuron disease, (b) age range of patients, (c) exclusion criteria, (d) stage and course of the disease, and, (e) number of patients entering and completing a therapeutic trial.

TYPE OF MOTOR NEURON DISEASE

Patients selected should have the classic (Charcot) form of ALS characterized by both upper and lower motor neuron signs as follows: (a) upper motor neuron signs, (increased muscle tone and hyperreflexia and/or a positive Babinski sign), (b) lower motor neuron signs, (weakness, muscle atrophy, and fasciculations). To be included in clinical trials, patients must have lower motor neuron signs, plus at least one additional upper motor neuron sign.

Each patient should have electrophysiological evidence of acute and chronic denervation. Muscle biopsy is not required, but , if biopsies have been done, results should be consistent with the diagnosis of ALS. Lumbar punctures should not be a requirement, but, if done, then the results should also be consistent with the diagnosis of ALS.

AGE OF THE PATIENTS

Patients under 21 should not be included in clinical trials, due to the high probability of their having an atypical course. Many published studies have had upper limits from 65 to 75, but exclusion criteria other than an upper age limit should be used.

EXCLUSION CRITERIA

Patients should be excluded from clinical trials if their presentation or course is atypical (Table 4-1). Absolute exclusion criteria should include sensory abnormalities, cerebellar involvement, neuro-ophthalmologic signs, or sphincter involvement. In essence, the clinical diagnosis of ALS should be unequivocal.

Progressive muscular atrophy (PMA), the purely lower motor neuron form of ALS, and primary lateral sclerosis (PLS), the purely upper motor neuron form of ALS, should be excluded from clinical trials, since there may be a variety of etiologies in both of these forms. PMA may be indistinguishable from late onset spinal muscular atrophy (Kugelberg-Welander), hexosaminidase-A deficiency, syphilitic amyotrophy, or even a scapuloperoneal syndrome. Patients presenting with PLS may also have diverse conditions including slowly progressive multiple sclerosis, adrenal leukodystrophy, and human T-lymphotrophic virus (HTLV-1) infection. Not only may the purely upper or lower motor neuron forms have diverse etiologies, but they also tend to have a better prognosis. Therefore, a clinical trial should not be complicated further by including forms of motor neuron disease that have an overall better prognosis than classic ALS.

If patients have either purely or predominantly bulbar signs with only minimal involvement of the limb muscles, they should be excluded from ALS clinical trials. Patients with advanced bulbar weakness to the point of being significantly malnourished should also be excluded, but those with a feeding tube who fit the other criteria for the study should be included.

Other forms of ALS that should be excluded are familial, those overlapping Alzheimer's dementia, or an amyotrophy with a multisystem disease. Other exclusion parameters include ALS secondary to plasma cell dyscrasia, hyper-

Table 4-1. *Exclusion Criteria*

Progressive muscular atrophy
Primary lateral sclerosis
Bulbar
Secondary forms of ALS
Too-advanced disease
Other significant medical illness
Medications

Table 4-2. *Types of MND Excluded from Clinical Trials*

Progressive muscular atrophy (PMA)
Kugelberg-Welander
Hexosaminidase A deficiency
Syphilitic amyotrophy
Scapuloperoneal syndrome
Primary lateral sclerosis
Multiple sclerosis
Adrenoleukodystrophy
HTLV-1 myelopathy
Secondary forms
Plasma cell dyscrasia
Hyperparathyroidism
Hyperthyroidism
Heavy metal poisoning
Irradiation
High-voltage electrical injury

parathyroidism or hyperthyroidism, association with intoxications (lead, aluminium, or mercury), or with physical agents (x-irradiation or high-voltage electrical injury) (Table 4-2).

Patients probably should not be permitted to take any central nervous system (CNS) depressant, psychoactive medication, antispasticity medication, or theophylline during a therapeutic trial, but this will vary depending on the pharmacological agent to be studied. If all medications had to be discontinued, there would be difficulty with patient recruitment, since symptomatic treatment is one of the main things that those taking care of ALS patients have to offer. To stop taking Lioresal, a tricyclic antidepressant, or atropine in order to enter a clinical study may lead to a worsening of the condition so that careful consideration should be given as to whether it is in the patient's best interest to take him off medications to make him eligible for a drug study.

There should be a reasonable expectation that the patients will be able to finish the study, so that an additional exclusion criterion should be based on pulmonary status. Anyone with a vital capacity of less than 60% of predicted at the start of the trial should not be included in a clinical trial, since there is a high probability that this patient will not survive 6 months (1). The patient should not have other diseases such as diabetes, hypertension requiring treatment, cardiac disease requiring treatment, severe asthma, or other significant impairment of respiratory function, significant endocrinopathy, or history of alcoholism or drug abuse.

In summary, the ideal patient for a therapeutic trial has classic ALS, with a progressive course and significant disability occurring within 2 years of symptoms. He should still be ambulatory, without other significant medical illness and on no medications. Bulbar dysfunction should be only minimal. Patients should be compliant in taking medication and reliable in attending follow-up evaluations.

STAGE AND COURSE OF THE DISEASE

The next and more difficult criteria to establish is where in the course of the disease a patient is, prior to the start of the study. Ideally, quantitative muscle strength testing (isometry) and perhaps also an ALS scale should be evaluated for a 3- to 6-month period prior to the start of the trial, as an important parameter in measuring the rate of progression. It would be optimal, in a drug trial, for equal numbers of patients receiving the active agents and the placebo to be as evenly distributed as possible with regard to their rate of deterioration. However, there may not be the opportunity to evaluate the patient for 3 to 6 months prior to the start of the trial. The investigator may have to construct, from the history and current examination, an assessment of the patient's rate of progression and the degree of involvement of the different pools of motor neurons (upper extremities, lower extremities, respiratory muscles, and bulbar muscles), and the rate of progression (classical, excessively fast, excessively slow). An alternative, depending on trial design, is a simple chronological criteria, such as the first symptom occurring within 3 years. To be sure that the course is progressive, significant deficits must occur within 2 years, and there should be no period longer that 3 months without progression. Regardless of the criteria used, a classical course and progression of ALS is essential for patient selection in clinical trials.

The patient should have significant weakness, but not so marked that there are too many muscle groups that are grade 3 or below in manual muscle testing, since this would greatly impair their ability to perform the required motor tests necessary to evaluate improvement with the drug. One way of establishing the criteria is to pick a number of muscles in which patients should have an analog MRC scale of greater than 3 and less than 5. If quantitative isometry is to be done, then a certain score could be established as part of the inclusion criteria. Patients who cannot ambulate should not be excluded on this criterion alone, if their overall muscle strength testing fits within the trial design. Rather than using just manual muscle testing results or isometry or a combination of the two, as inclusion criteria, an alternative is a certain score on an ALS scale, such as the Norris scale (2), Tuft's quantitative neuromuscular exam (3),the ALS severity scale (4), or perhaps a composite scale, as yet undesigned.

NUMBER OF PATIENTS IN THE TRIAL

The type of study is also important in patient selection. In general, a crossover study is preferred by patients, because all patients will eventually get the active drug (5). This is an important issue in regard to recruitment, since patients are more likely to join a trial in which they have 100% chance of getting the drug as compared to a parallel study in which they have only a 50% chance. An inducement in a parallel trial is to give the drug to everyone who received placebo after the trial has ended.

There are fewer dropouts in a crossover trial because , if deterioration occurs in the first period of the trial, patients will stay in the trial in order to obtain the other substance, which they hope will be more effective. In a parallel study, continuing deterioration may well lead patients to drop out and seek alternative treatment (6). An additional advantage of the crossover trial is that less patients are required than in a parallel study. A crossover study is more efficient in determining how big a difference the treatment makes, since differences within the same patient are often more significant than differences between groups of patients.

In considering patients to be included in a clinical trial, the entire list of ALS patients is reviewed and those with exclusion criteria eliminated from the list. Depending on the design of the protocol, the number of patients available will be reduced by 33%–66%. Subsequent recruitment should be successful in the range of 50%–75%. The number of patients that actually complete the trial will also vary, depending on the design protocol.

An example is the Levamisole Trial conducted by Dr. Olarte and Shaffer at Columbia Presbyterian from 1978 to 1981 (7). They began with patients with a clinical diagnosis of ALS, but in order to be eligible for the trial, a Norris score of greater than 45 was required. Of the original 232 patients, 122 had a score of over 45. Of this number only 59 consented to the randomized trial.

Less than 50% of the eligible patients entered the trial because they did not want placebo, possible side-effects, monthly visits, or any experimental treatment. Most patients refused to enter because of the double-blind design of the trial, even though it was a crossover study. Of 59 patients who entered the trial, 30 withdrew, due to progression of the disease without any apparent effectiveness of the drug. Over 3 years, only 19 of 118 possible candidates completed the 1-year trial.

In another trial, which was a short-term (16 day) parallel design, high-dose, subcutaneous TRH study at Henry Ford Hospital, there were a variety of categories to describe the patient selection process. Of a list of 100 ALS patients, 15 were eligible for the trial, and 9 entered with 6 declining. Thirty-one percent had too-advanced disease, including 9% on ventilators. Other major categories of exclusion were too-advanced bulbar disease (12%), concurrent medical illness requiring medication (15%), and either entirely lower motor neuron findings or an atypical course (17%) (Table 4-3).

Patient recruitment needs to be enhanced. There are too many clinical trials in which a large number of patients that fit the criteria do not elect to enter the study. The key issues are a strict definition of ALS, the effect of medications and other medical illnesses on the study, the stage and course of the disease, the age and life expectancy due to pulmonary status, and the type of drug trial.

Table 4-3. *Patient Selection (n=100)*

Criteria	Percent
Included in study	9
Declined	6
Too advanced (ventilator)	32(9)
Bulbar	12
Atypical	16
Medications	14
Too strong	7
Deceased	4

The use of uniform criteria for patient selection in all therapeutic trials would allow investigators to compare results in a much more efficient fashion. At present, it is extremely difficult to compare clinical trials in which patients with lower motor neuron forms of ALS and bulbar ALS are included in one trial and excluded in another. Similarly, clinical trials should be designed so that results in patients with long-term survival are not compared to patients who have a very rapid course. The use of uniform criteria would greatly expand the concept of multicenter trials, and allow the individual investigator flexibility in evaluating a variety of pharmacological agents and use different forms of testing patients and evaluating the results.

REFERENCES

1. Küther G, Struppler A, Lipinski HG. Therapeutic trials in ALS: the design of a protocol. In: Cosi V, Kato AC, Parlette W, Pinelli P, Poloni M, eds. *Amyotrophic lateral sclerosis: therapeutic, psychological and research aspects.* New York: Plenum Press, 1987;265-76.
2. Norris FH, Calanchini PR, Fallat RJ, et al. The administration of guanidine in amyotrophic lateral sclerosis. *Neurology* 1971; 24:721-8.
3. Andres PL, Hedlund W, Finison L, et al. Quantitative motor assessment in amyotrophic lateral sclerosis. *Neurology* 1986; 36:937-41.
4. Hillel AD, Miller RM, McDonald E, et al. ALS severity scale. In: Tsubaki T, Yase Y, eds, *Amyotrophic lateral sclerosis: recent advances in research and treatment.* Amsterdam: Elsevier, 1988:247-52.
5. Rose FC, Clinical trials in motor neuron disease (MND). In: Tsubaki T, Yase Y, eds, *Amyotrophic lateral sclerosis: recent advances in research and treatment.* Amsterdam: Elsevier, 1988;281-5.
6. Shaffer SQ, Olarte MR. Methodological considerations for clinical trials in motor neuron disease. In: LP Rowland, ed, *Human motor neuron disease.* New York: Raven Press, 1982;559-65. (Advances in neurology; vol 36.)
7. Olarte M, Shaffer SQ. Levamisole is ineffective in the treatment of amyotrophic lateral sclerosis. *Neurology* 1985; 35:1063-6.

Amyotrophic Lateral Sclerosis,
edited by F. Clifford Rose.
Demos Publications, New York © 1990.

5

Should Amyotrophic Lateral Sclerosis Trials Not Be Placebo Controlled?

Lars-Olof Ronnevi

Department of Clinical Neurology,
Karolinska Sjukhuset, Stockholm, Sweden

In 1980 Festoff and Crigger (1) reported a survey of 38 amyotrophic lateral sclerosis (ALS) treatment trials up to that time. According to a set of criteria (Table 5-1), they concluded that no less than 36 of theses studies had been technically unsatisfactory. Although the situation has changed to some degree since then, their findings are a criticism against clinical researchers working in the ALS field, especially because their criteria for an adequate study design are generally accepted by the scientific community and most national drug control administrations. Thirty-four of the studies reviewed were criticized because they lacked untreated or placebo-treated control groups, so there is a need to analyze the reasons why clinical researchers have been reluctant to include placebo treatment in therapeutic trials of ALS. This is an issue that has been addressed by different authors (3–6), and there may be situations in which we should consider alternatives to a placebo-based design.

PSYCHOLOGICAL PROBLEMS

A basic problem with including placebo treatment in ALS is obviously the psychological reaction to, and the acceptance of, this form of treatment by the patient. Placebo medication, by definition, means treatment with an agent lacking pharmacological effect, and its nature and use, whether openly or masked, must be explained to the patient as part of the informed consent preceding a trial (7). Anyone confronted with the clinical features of ALS will agree that patients with this disease are in a very special psychological situation with regard to placebo trials when compared with patients who have most other

Table 5-1 *Criteria for Evaluating Clinical Trials in Amyotrophic Lateral Sclerosis According to Festoff and Crigger (1)*

Clinical plus electromyographic muscle-biopsy diagnosis
Randomized drug therapy
Inclusion of control group taking placebo
Double-blind study
Standardized treatment for both groups
Objective measurements of follow-up evaluation and analysis of results

diseases that equal ALS in prognosis. There is a monotonous deterioration of mobility and communication ability and virtually no hope for an arrest of progress. Mortality is close to 100% in an easily foreseeable future and no remedy, even one delaying the course, is offered by the medical profession. This fact is experienced by a person who has intact mental and emotional capacities throughout the disease course. When a person in this discouraging situation is offered participation in a treatment trial, the possible effect of an active drug owes the one and only chance to escape an otherwise inevitable, disabling course ending in death. It is not surprising that the first fear expressed by many patients when confronted with the prospect of a treatment trial is the use of placebo medication.

Theoretically, the active drug in a trial is of no better therapeutic value than the control regimen until proven by the study to be conducted, but this is an intellectual point of view when considered by the patient, from whose view–point the physician announces a high degree of unspoken confidence in the active drug simply by being prepared to conduct the trial

FALL-OFF AND CROSS-CONTAMINATION

The difficulty that arises when a significant number of patients disapprove, openly or not, of the possibility of placebo treatment can technically be counteracted by linking enrollment in the study to the study design. In so doing there is the risk of exploiting the patient's possible fears that a refusal to participate would have negative effects on other aspects of his or her medical attention, but we also introduce significant sources of error in the interpretation of the forthcoming results. If a commercially available drug is tested, patients may not refuse participation in the study but agree to enrollment to please the physician, and secure the active drug from some other source. This form of cross-contamination of a study is difficult to trace. If the patient cannot get hold of the active drug outside the study, suspected exposure to placebo reduces the motivation for continuing medication for longer periods.

An alternative to this situation is to accept a possibly high degree of primary fall-off by offering open treatment with the active drug to patients unwilling to accept the placebo design, to use a crossover design or both of these measures (3). The value of crossover is reduced in studies in which a long observation period is required, which is necessary as long as our evaluation systems merely monitor secondary effects of loss of motor neurons, whether linear or not (8,9), rather than the primary disease process itself. In a crossover design study, patients who have experienced a beneficial effect from the first regimen offered, whether based on a real therapeutic effect or not, are reluctant to switch over to the second drug (6).

NONRANDOM NONCOMPLIANCE

The placebo-related types of noncompliance are of special importance because they cannot be supposed to occur at random in a group of ALS patients. In a progressive disease such as ALS they are more likely to occur in patients experiencing a rapid deterioration. An open treatment alternative is more likely to be demanded by the same category of patients. Both a nonrandom noncompliance and primary fall-off reduce the chances to detect smaller treatment differences, including both positive treatment effects and unrecognized adverse effects of the medication (2).

In addition to the ethical aspects, the use of placebo treatment in ALS trials is associated with a number of difficult technical problems. Common reasons for criticism of inadequate trial designs in ALS or any serious disorder is the risk of awakening false hopes among patients and relatives, and the fear that inadequate protocols or evaluations would delay the detection of true benefits form a certain drug and delay the availability of effective treatment to the patients.

All these risks also apply to a double-blind placebo-based trial and may even be amplified by the increased impact of this kind of study on the medical profession. The placebo treatment problem may be among the most important of potential sources of error in a clinical ALS trial together with, for example, inconsistencies in diagnosis and subgrouping of the patients. The handling of the placebo-associated sources of error requires a marked extension of study groups (2).

ALTERNATIVE STRATEGIES FOR PRELIMINARY STUDIES

The problems discussed mean that a decision to go for a placebo-based evaluation must rest on solid preliminary evidence of a positive treatment effect, and such studies should preferably not be initiated until we are willing to provide the resources necessary to provide conclusive results.

What are the alternatives in the more preliminary stages of treatment evaluation? Independently repeated studies with, for example, blinded multiparametrical evaluation of disease progress, may well be adequate for detecting

Table 5-2. *Reports of Mean or Median Survival Time in Amyotrophic Lateral Sclerosis*

Reference	Mean/median survival (mo)
Friedman and Freedman (12)	34.0 (mean)
Brain et al. (13)	32.0 (mean)
Vejjajiva et al. (14)	36.0 (mean)
Bonduelle (15)	34.5 (mean)
Kristensen and Melgaard (16)	31.2 (median)
Juergens et al. (17)	22.5 (median)
Forsgren et al. (18)	33.6 (median)
Caroscio et al. (19)	60.1 (median)

a hypothetical ideal ALS treatment, i.e., one that gives complete arrest of the disease process in the majority of patients; for example, evaluation of penicillin in bacterial infection did not involve a single untreated control (10).

An additional possibility for preliminary study is a treatment that acts on a continuous or ordinal laboratory parameter associated with the disease process in ALS. In such a situation, the degree of response of the parameter to a certain treatment can be correlated with disease progress during treatment. We have used this principle in a recent study on the correlation between the clinical progress rate in ALS patients and the lowering of cytotoxic plasma activity induced by immunosuppression (11).

It may also be possible to use survival time in preliminary treatment evaluation as compared with untreated controls, but with respect to diagnostic criteria and clinical subgrouping of reference as well as treatment groups. Evidence of the possible usefulness of this approach is derived from the striking uniformity in mean or median survival in many reports from different geographical areas and times (Table 5-2).

STRATEGIES FOR CLINICAL TRIALS

As judged from present clues to etiology and pathogenesis in ALS, it is likely that the first effective ALS treatment will be one that slows down, rather than arrests, the disease progress in most patients. We may end up in a situation in which a final and conclusive evaluation of a certain ALS treatment is absolutely critical and impossible to achieve without a complete clinical trial, including placebo treatment. When the decision to undertake such a trial is made, there is great ethical and scientific responsibility. To justify the psychological trauma caused to individual patients by this study design, the beneficial effects from the treatment should not be clinically self-evident but should be strongly suggested by previous studies with an alternative design. For the sake of validity it is essential that a study group of adequate size is used and it is absolutely critical that we keep to agreed diagnostic and classification criteria. To ensure this, multicenter approaches should be seriously considered, particularly because there is a need to come up with an answer in the shortest possible time.

Acknowledgment: The support from the Swedish Medical Research Council (proj. 5178) and the Karolinska Institute is gratefully acknowledged.

REFERENCES

1. Festoff B., Crigger NJ. Therapeutic trials in amyotrophic lateral sclerosis: a review. In: Mulder DW, ed. *The diagnosis and treatment of amyotrophic lateral sclerosis.* Boston: Houghton Mifflin, 1980: 337–66.
2. Meinert CL, Tonascia S. *Clinical trials. Design, conduct and analysis.* New York: Oxford University Press, 1986.
3. Tyler HR. Double-blind study of modified neurotoxin in motor neuron disease. *Neurology* 1979; 29:77–81.
4. Tyler HR. Commentary. In: Mulder DW, ed. *The diagnosis and treatment of amyotrophic lateral sclerosis.* Boston: Houghton Mifflin, 1980: 367–8.
5. Festoff BW. Approaches to modern therapeutic clinical trials in ALS. In: Clifford Rose F, ed. *Research progress in motor neurone disease.* London: Pitman, 1984: 432–42.
6. Rose FC. Clinical trials in motor neurone disease. In: Tsubaki T., Yase Y, ed. *Amyotrophic lateral sclerosis. Recent advances in research and treatment. Excerpta Medica International Congress Series 769.* Amsterdam: Elsevier, 1988: 281–5.
7. U.S. Office for Protection from Research Risks. Protection of human subjects. Title 45: Public Welfare, Part 46. Bethesda: National Institutes of Health, 1983.
8. Munsat TL, Andres PL, Finison L, et al. The natural history of motorneuron loss in amyotrophic lateral sclerosis. *Neurology* 1988; 38:409–13.
9. Küther G. Lipinski H-G. Computer simulation of neuron degeneration in motor neuron disease. In: Tsubaki T, Yase Y, eds. *Amyotrophic lateral sclerosis. Recent advances in research and treatment. Excerpta Medica International Series 729.* Amsterdam: Elsevier, 1988: 131–7.
10. Keefer CS, Blake FG, Marshall EK Jr, et al. Penicillin in the treatment of infections: a report of 500 cases. *J Am Med Assoc* 1943; 122:1217–24.
11. Ronnevi LO, Conradi S. Cytotoxic activity in ALS-patients. In: Tsubaki T, Yase Y, eds. *Amyotrophic lateral sclerosis. Recent advances in research and treatment. Excerpta Medica International Congress Series 769.* Amsterdam: Elsevier, 1988:149–54.
12. Friedman AP, Freedman D. Amyotrophic lateral sclerosis. *J Nerv Ment Dis* 1950; 3:1–18.
13. Brain WR, Croft P., Wilkinson M. The course and outcome of motor neuron disease. In: Norris FH, Kurland LT, eds. *Motor neuron diseases.* New York: Grune and Stratton, 1967: 22–8.
14. Vejjajiva A, Foster JB, Miller H. Motor neuron disease. A clinical study. *J Neurol Sci* 1967; 4:299–314.
15. Bonduelle M. Amyotrophic lateral sclerosis. In: Vinken PJ, Bruyn GW, eds. *Handbook of clinical neurology,* vol 22. Amsterdam: Elsevier, 1975: 281–9.
16. Kristensen O, Melgaard B. Motor neuron disease. Prognosis and epidemiology. *Acta Neurol Scand* 1977; 56:299–308.

17. Juergens SM, Kurland LT, Okayaki PH, et al. ALS in Rochester, Minnesota, 1925–1977. *Neurology* 1980; 30:463–70.
18. Forsgren L, Almay BGL, Holmgren X, et al. Epidemiology of motor neuron disease in northern Sweden. *Acta Neurol Scand* 1983; 68:20–9.
19. Caroscio JT, Calhoun WF, Yahr MD. Prognostic factors in motor neurone disease: a prospective study of longevity. In: Clifford Rose F, ed. *Research progress in motor neurone disease.* London: Pitman, 1984: 34–43.

Amyotrophic Lateral Sclerosis,
edited by F. Clifford Rose.
Demos Publications, New York © 1990.

6

Influence of Compliance and Other Human Factors on Treatment Trials

Richard Alan Smith, Sherri Jacoby, Barry Festoff, Lori Peterson, Schlomo Melmed, Gabriella Molnar, Barry Sherman, and James Frane

Center for Neurologic Study, San Diego, California; Kansas City Veterans Administration Medical Center, Kansas City, Missouri; Cedar Sinai Hospital, Los Angeles, California; and Genentech Corporation, San Francisco, California, U.S.A.

The experimental treatment of amyotrophic lateral sclerosis (ALS) offers the possibility of revolutionizing the therapy of a presently incurable disease and of advancing knowledge of the etiology of a poorly understood pathologic process. Without a known cause,the rationale for treatment is highly speculative, but the will to treat is understandable given the opportunities that have accompanied the general advance of medicine and science. In clinical trials, it is assumed that a highly motivated patient and physician have faithfully followed the prescribed protocol and that the data faithfully reflect the optimal test of the experimental hypothesis. Unfortunately, a number of human factors confound the best intentions of clinical research.

One of the most neglected of clinical trial variables is the issue of compliance. This, by definition, occurs when either the patient or physician fail to follow the protocol or therapeutic regimen. Under ideal circumstances, all of the requirements of a treatment trial would be thoroughly controlled, but in practice this is not always feasible in studies with human subjects.

Physicians generally overestimate compliance and are unable to discern which of their patients will exhibit it. Speculating on the origin for this ignorance, some have suggested a psychological cause (DiMatteo, 1982). Convinced of their authority and status, physicians may fail to recognize behavior that does not reaffirm their beliefs. There are other equally plausible explanations. In some instances, physicians are probably unaware of the naivete of human behavior; committed as they are to medicine as a discipline, it is easy to accept that patients are guided by the same principles.

Hippocrates, commenting on patient behavior, advised physicians to "keep a watch also on the faults of the patients, which often make them lie about the taking of things prescribed." Although intent is difficult to discern, it is clear from numerous studies that there are marked discrepancies between patient reports of compliance and fact. It has been suggested that misrepresentations are rationalized by patients in an effort to please physicians or to avoid rejection by them. In some instances, the patient has misunderstood instructions, compliance being a product of the transaction between patient and physician (Stone, 1979). If viewed exclusively as a patient problem, noncompliance, in Stone's view, becomes a moral problem. On this basis, the patient is unlikely to accept culpability for failing to adhere to a medical regimen, but if compliance is seen as a shared responsibility, then patients are more amenable to accept and critically evaluate their role in the treatment process. Obviously, this process is facilitated in the context of a caring physician/patient relationship, which places demands on the physician who may need to bridge differences in social status, education, or cultural identity.

The character of the physician's response to compliance reports obviously influences patient willingness to enter a dialogue with their practitioner. Terse or desultory comments are unlikely to elicit complete and truthful replies, but the interviewer can influence patients in more subtle ways. Response bias occurs when certain classes of behavior are reinforced or discouraged.Doctors may unwittingly signal that they would prefer not hearing about some aspects of the patient's history. Responses that reinforce recall (that is the kind of information I need to know, etc.) are, on the contrary, likely to increase reporting. If demands are made on memory, it may be useful to provide instructions to the patient so that they will appreciate the character of information that they will be asked to recall in later interviews.

ASSESSMENT OF COMPLIANCE

A number of means have been used to measure compliance, none of which are ideal (Feinstein and Ransohoff, 1976). Patient logs rely on self-reporting to determine medication use, but this type of information can be supplemented with an actual count of the medication dispensed. Monitoring the drug directly or indirectly in blood or other biological fluids offers direct confirmation of compliance but is not foolproof. Each of these assessment modes can be flawed. Patient compliance reports, for example, are often considerably inflated when independently validated. Comparing self-reports with real-time monitoring (Kass et al., 1986) revealed a wide disparity between these measures of compliance. Patients who reported taking their medication 95% or more of the time often showed a compliance rate of 45% or less when monitored electronically.

With pill counts, even when the proper amount of medication is taken it is impossible to reconstruct the dosage regimen. A recent study of the pattern of use of a topical ophthalmological drug prescribed at six-hour intervals found a wide variation in the dosage schedules (Kass et al., 1986). Medication was often taken long before or after the prescribed time. When efficacy of treatment depends on proper dosing, it is clear that compliance with the prescribed regimen is an important treatment variable.

Laboratory determination of drugs or metabolites may be hampered by the short half-life of the active ingredient. Under these circumstances, the pattern of drug usage can only be inferred for the interval immediately preceding the test. In most instances,the placebo cannot be measured. To counter this problem, the use of a marker is not without problems (Baron, 1984). Before the start of the trial, screening needs to be conducted to establish the validity of the test, and the range of values to indicate compliance set. In some instances, cross-reactivity with nonprescribed medication can spuriously elevate laboratory values, resulting in false positives; this can incorrectly suggest drop-ins to the trial, i.e., a patient who is supposedly taking placebo seeming to receive the active drug.

PROTROPIN STUDY

To ascertain the variables which influence outcome in a treatment trial, we analyzed data from a recently completed treatment trial that incorporated contemporary concepts of trial design. Seventy-seven patients (42 men) were enrolled in a double-blind placebo-controlled trial. The test substance was a genetically engineered hormone. At serial intervals, the course of ALS was monitored using Tufts Quantitative Neuromuscular Examination (TQNE). A number of unique characteristics of this trial provide the opportunity to assess human factors in a contemporary setting. It was initially intended to recruit 80 patients equally between three centers, enrolling all of the patients at one time. Due to the stringent exclusion criteria this proved to be impossible, and ultimatelyfour separate cohorts were enrolled at two-month intervals. A disproportionate number of patients were enrolled at two of the three centers. Four months into the trial patients were queried as to their attitude toward the staff and the trial. At the outset, as expected, there was uniform appreciation on the part of the subjects toward the staff. Commenting on the actions and behavior of the staff that might be expected to influence patient attitudes, it was found that nurses were thought to communicate better than physicians did but that the latter were thought to be more available when help was needed. However, when called on,physicians did not always respond to the patient's needs (Table 6-1).

Table 6-1. *Data from Patient Questionnaire Administered to Subjects in an Experimental Treatment Trial of Amyotrophic Lateral Sclerosis*

	Good (%)	Adequate (%)	Poor (%)	No comment (%)
Communication				
Physician		85	13	2
Nurse		96	4	
Availability				
Physician		98		2
Nurse		73[a]		27
Response to Needs				
Physician	72	4	2	22

[a] One center 25%.

The ultimate effect, if any, of these attitudes on patient participation is a matter for further study but the responses did signal an early problem with staff compliance at one center. As the study proceeded it became clear that one staff member failed to comply with procedures in the protocol. These departures were thought to be serious enough to warrant a change of staff.

Age,surprisingly, did not seem to influence the decision to stay in or drop out of the trial. However, mortality was higher in the older age group. Unexpectedly the neuromuscular status of the patient at the time of enrollment in the trial did not influence the dropout, but deterioration of arm strength did correlate with withdrawal from the study. Persons who rapidly lost use of their arms were most likely to drop out.

At the end of the twelve month study, only twenty-six of the initial seventy-seven patients remained. In short, about a third of the patients completed the trial, a fourth died and the remainder withdrew. Losses of this magnitude and greater are common to ALS trials, which has been commented on by Olarte, who observed a 55% attrition rate at 1 year in a trial of ALS with levamisole (Olarte, 1982).

Because growth hormone raises the level of IGF-1 in growth-deficient children, it was decided to monitor the levels of this hormone in patients enrolled in the trial, as a guide to compliance. As can be noted from Fig. 6-1, most of the patients receiving growth hormone experienced an increase in IGF-1,whereas there was little change in patients receiving placebo.However, the data illustrate one of the problems involved when an attempt is made to measure compliance with a biological marker.Some of the patients were found to have relatively high IGF-1 levels before treatment, whereas others who received placebo showed an increase in IGF-1 values.

Table 6-2. *Effect of Compliance on Sample Size*

Patients who comply (%)	Placebo success rate (%)	Treatment group success rate (%)	Group size
100	40	58	131
90	40	57	148
70	40	55	195
50	40	53	267

IMPACT OF NONCOMPLIANCE ON TRIAL DESIGN

Reviewing the impact of compliance on the requirements for conduct of controlled trials, Schectman and Gordon calculated that noncompliant patients in a cholesterol study received only 35% of the therapeutic effect of control patients (K.B. Schectman and M. E. Gordon, unpublished data, 1986). Extrapolating from the data, they determined hypothetical sample sizes for randomized controlled trials with customary levels of power (.9) and significance (.05). In these estimates they defined a compliant patient as one who took 80% of their medication at the prescribed schedule. It can be seen from these extrapolations that the sample size requirements increase dramatically as the compliance rate falls, increasing approximately 2-1/2-fold as the compliance falls to 50% (Table 6-2).

Noncompliance can also exert a major effect when it is different in the treatment and placebo groups. This is usually due to side-effects that affect compliance. Again, analyzing data from the cholesterol study, Schectman and Gordon calculated that disparity in compliance rates greatly affects the size of the groups required in placebo-controlled trials. This occurred because compliance in the placebo limb of their trial was 67% versus 51% in the treatment limb.

STRATEGIES TO INFLUENCE COMPLIANCE

Before the Trial

If efficacy is an important goal of the trial, it is necessary to enroll a maximal number of compliant patients. Efficacy is a measure of the therapeutic effect in patients who take medication as intended, whereas effectiveness is a measure of the therapeutic effect in a representative population. To maximize efficacy it may be useful to incorporate a prerandomization run-in period. Patients who do not tolerate medication or who are noncompliant can then be deemed ineligible. In a recent trial involving physicians, approximately 30% of potential

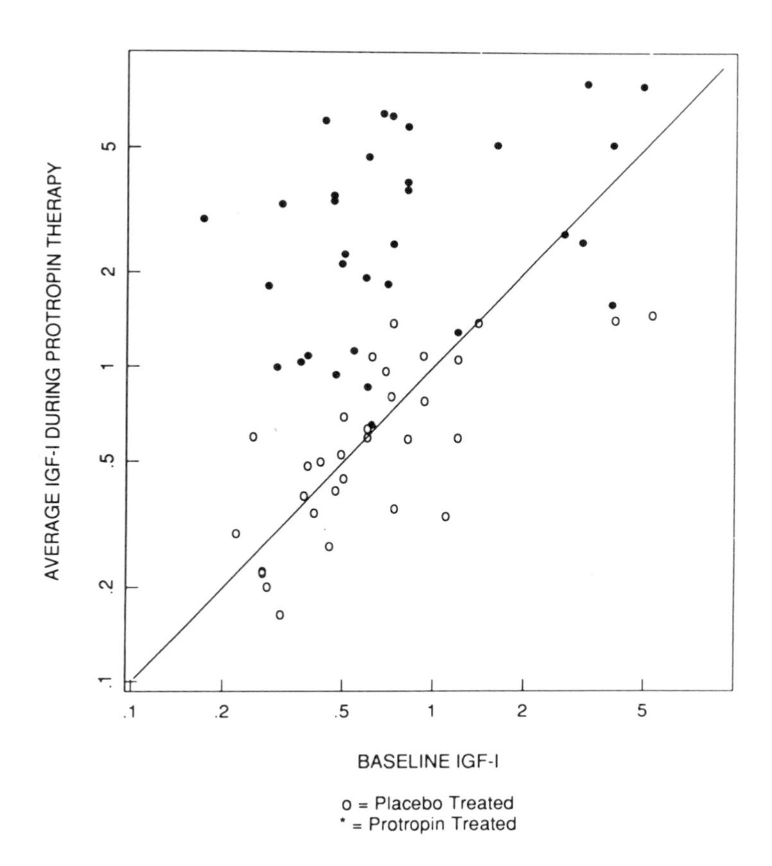

FIG. 6-1. IGF-1 values (units per milliliter) are plotted at baseline and during treatment. The diagonal indicates "no change" in IGF-1.

participants were excluded after the run-in period. Those who went on to complete the trial were thought to have maintained a relatively high compliance rate - greater than 80% (Belanger, et al., 1988).

Although run-in favorably influences compliance, it does have disadvantages. Unwittingly, subjects in trials with active drug controls could prefer one treatment over another. Furthermore,selection may not be random, because factors segregating compliance such as age could result in underrepresentation of subjects in one limb of the trial. Trials with a run-in feature may overestimate effectiveness and underestimate efficacy because the trial participants do not fully represent patients in the general population. In short, the use of run-in requires caution.

During the Trial

Although ALS patients are highly motivated to participate in trials, their commitment often lags as the trial proceeds. There are three obvious causes for this attitudinal change. With disease progression it is easy to lose faith in the investigation, and as disability increases it becomes burdensome to meet the needs of the study as well as personal needs.Finally, patients are tempted to abandon the trials for other treatment. This occurs when they hear about other trials or when they choose unconventional treatment.

Assuming normal bonding between investigator, staff, and patient,there are a number of things that can be done to enhance compliance. Most of these involve improved communication (Friedman, et al., 1985). During recruitment it is advisable to stress the study rather than the drug. Overemphasis on the drug encourages participants to obtain treatment outside of the trial.There are instances in which patients will test their medication to determine whether it is the active or placebo formulary.

Although there are no substitutes for a good relationship between staff and patient, several formal steps can be implemented to encourage compliance in treatment trials. The following have been employed in some studies: (a) literature—study brochure,newsletter; (b) telephone and mail contact; (c) drug dispensers;(d) reminders; and (e) contracts.

Although the impact of these on compliance has not been tested,it is certain from research that patients interpret the failure of physicians to address compliance in their visits as a lack of concern on the part of the caregiver in this issue. Investigating compliance in a general practice setting, it has been found that physician behavior can greatly influence medication usage by patients (Di Matteo and Di Nicola, 1982). Historical information provided to physicians was more complete and truthful when compliance was monitored.

CONCLUSIONS

Treatment trials, especially those involving patients with incurable diseases, should make allowances for human factors that often complicate the execution of clinical research. In some respects one can see parallels between the behavior of patients and physician/scientists who comprise the ALS research community. Both groups are sometimes swept up in the enthusiasm of the moment for this or that therapeutic claim. In ALS treatment trials there are large losses due to death and to dropout. This imposes special constraints that cannot be ignored. Few treatment trials of ALS make note of these factors in reporting their results, presumably because they were not assessed or because investigators have chosen to ignore this aspect of trial design (Festoff and Crigger, 1979). It is not clear whether attention to these details will ultimately prove important to identifying a therapy for ALS, but it is reasonable to assume that the cause of ALS is well served by improving the quality of treatment trials.

Acknowledgment: This work was supported by the Joseph Drown Foundation, the Thagard Foundation, the Muscular Dystrophy Association, and Genetech Corporation.

REFERENCES

1. Baron JA, Compliance issues/biological markers. In: Sestilli MA,ed. *Chemoprevention clinical trials: problems and solutions.* Bethesda: NCI, 1985.
2. Belanger C, et al. Preliminary report: findings from the aspirin component of the ongoing physicians' health study. *New Engl J Med* 1988;318:262–4.
3. Di Matteo MR, Di Nicola DD. *Achieving patient compliance: the psychology of the medical practitioner's role.* New York: Pergamon Press, 1982.
4. Festoff BW, Crigger NJ. Therapeutic trials in amyotrophic lateral sclerosis: a review. In: Mulder DW, ed. *The diagnosis and treatment of amyotrophic lateral sclerosis.* Boston: Houghton Mifflin, 1980:337–69.
5. Feinstein AR, Ransohoff DF, Problems of compliance as a source of bias in data analysis. In: Lasagna L, ed. *Patient compliance.* 1976.
6. Friedman FM, Furberg CD, De Mets DL. *Fundamentals of clinical trials.* Massachusetts: Publishing Science Group, 1985.
7. Kass MA, Gordon M, Meltzer DW. Can ophthalmologists correctly identify patients defaulting from pilocarpine therapy? *Am J Ophthalmol* 1986b; 101:524–30.
8. Kass MA, Meltzer DW, et al. Compliance with topical pilocarpine treatment. *Am J Ophthalmol* 1986a; 101:515–23.
9. Olarte MR, Therapeutic trials in amyotrophic lateral sclerosis. In: Rowland LP, ed. *Human motor neuron diseases.* New York: Raven Press,1982:555–7.
10. Stone GC, Cohen F, Adler NE. *Health psychology.* San Francisco: Jossey Bass, 1979.

Amyotrophic Lateral Sclerosis,
edited by F. Clifford Rose.
Demos Publications, New York © 1990.

7

Measurements of Muscle Strength

Russell J. M. Lane

International ALS Research Group on Methodological Problems in ALS Trials, Charing Cross Hospital, London, England

Weakness and fatigue are the cardinal symptoms in most neuromuscular disorders, yet the techniques and problems involved in the quantitation of muscle strength and the detection of significant strength changes during treatment have received surprisingly little attention, at least in the neurological literature. This is to some extent a reflection of the difficulties involved in such measurements, because the "observed strength" of a muscle or muscle group at any time depends essentially on an interaction between the subject being tested,the observer, and the instruments and equipment used for the measurements, and is subject to volitional factors and other variables. Nevertheless, detailed studies over many years have shown that careful, standardized techniques can provide quantitative information with surprisingly small intra- and inter-observer variations (1–5). Muscle strength measurements are of particular importance in trials of treatment in amyotrophic lateral sclerosis, for which there is no independent index or marker of disease activity or progression beyond clinical observation.

Quantitative strength studies are important in neuromuscular disease research if we are not to miss potentially important *biological* effects of treatment, irrespective of any immediate functional significance. For example, there have been several published trials of plasma exchange (PE) in Guillain-Barré syndrome, and results have varied in terms of the impact of treatment on morbidity. The first studies (6, 7) failed to demonstrate that PE had a beneficial effect, but subsequent trials suggested that PE undertaken early in the course of the disease resulted in earlier remission and less morbidity, particularly in terms of time spent in high-dependency units and duration of inpatient care (8–10).

Surprisingly, none of these studies employed quantitative strength assessments, but rather responses to treatment were judged using ordinal rating

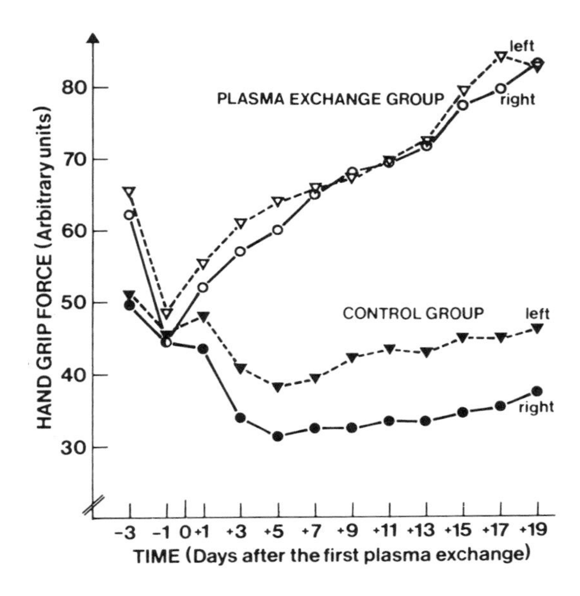

FIG. 7-1. Changes in hand-grip force in 14 plasma exchange and 15 conservatively treated patients with Guillain-Barré syndrome. [Reproduced from Färkkilä et al. (11) with permission.]

scales and subjective factors, such as time spent in the hospital. However, in a recent single-center study (11), serial hand-grip measurements were used in addition to functional assessments. Patients undergoing PE showed a marked improvement in distal muscle strength compared with the control group (Fig. 7-1); it was evident that the treatment had a positive biological effect, at least in terms of strength of the muscle groups studied, although no overall functional benefit could be demonstrated.

DEFINITIONS AND UNITS OF MEASUREMENT

Strength is a physiological concept described in terms of a physical parameter: the *force* exerted by a muscle or muscle group. *Isometric force* is generated by a muscle when no work is done by the contraction, i.e., when no displacement of the load occurs. This is sometimes referred to as *static strength,* or *maximal voluntary contraction,* and should strictly be described in units of mass (kilograms or pounds),although it is frequently quoted in newtons, the physiological unit of force (Table 7-1). When muscle contracts *isotonically,* it exerts a constant force throughout the contraction; strength measured under such conditions is often referred to as *dynamic strength.* The contraction may

Table 7-1. *Definitions and Units*

Definition	Units
Strength — linear/rotational	Kilograms, newtons[a]
Work — force x displacement	Joules, kilopond meter[b]
Power — rate of working	Watts (joules per second)
Effort — work x time	Kilopond-meter-second or minute

[a] Newton is a unit of force, i.e., mass x acceleration, kilogram-meter per second squared.
[b] Kilopond is the physiological unit of force. One kilopond is the gravitational force on a mass of 1kg.

be *concentric*, the muscle shortening to overcome and displace an external load; or *eccentric*, by contracting against an external force that tends to lengthen the muscle. Strength measured under these conditions is thus described in units of *work* (joules, kilopond-meters, or foot-pounds), being the product of the force and the displacement.

Experiments have shown that measurements of isometric,concentric, and eccentric strength of a muscle group are highly correlated in any individual, but that concentric strength is consistently less, and eccentric strength greater, than isometric strength (12). The quantitative differences in dynamic strength measurements depend on the rate of movement, and may be ±40% of the isometric strength (12). For this reason, recent research methods have concentrated on isometric measurements, or have employed the newer concept of *isokinetic dynamometry*. This allows measurement of work done by individual muscle groups over a specified range of motion performed at a constant rate that can be varied over a wide range, allowing assessment of dynamic strength, efficiency, and fatigue characteristics at various rates of working (13).

SELECTION OF APPROPRIATE MUSCLE STRENGTH TESTS

No one test can fully define muscle strength, and tests have to be selected or designed with regard to the disease under investigation and the particular questions to be answered. The three factors to be considered in any strength-measurement technique are the *validity* of the test, with regard to the pathogenesis of the disease, the *sensitivity* of the test to change during disease progression or in response to treatment,and the *reliability* of the procedure in terms of reproducibility in intra- and inter-observer studies. A combination of static and dynamic measurements together with functional rating scales will usually be employed, but observed improvements in functional scores during treatment may be due to complex adaptive motor behavior rather than to significant biological alterations or changes in the fundamental pathogenetic process. Conversely, recovery of dynamic strength and endurance can lag behind improvements in static muscle strength during treatment in some

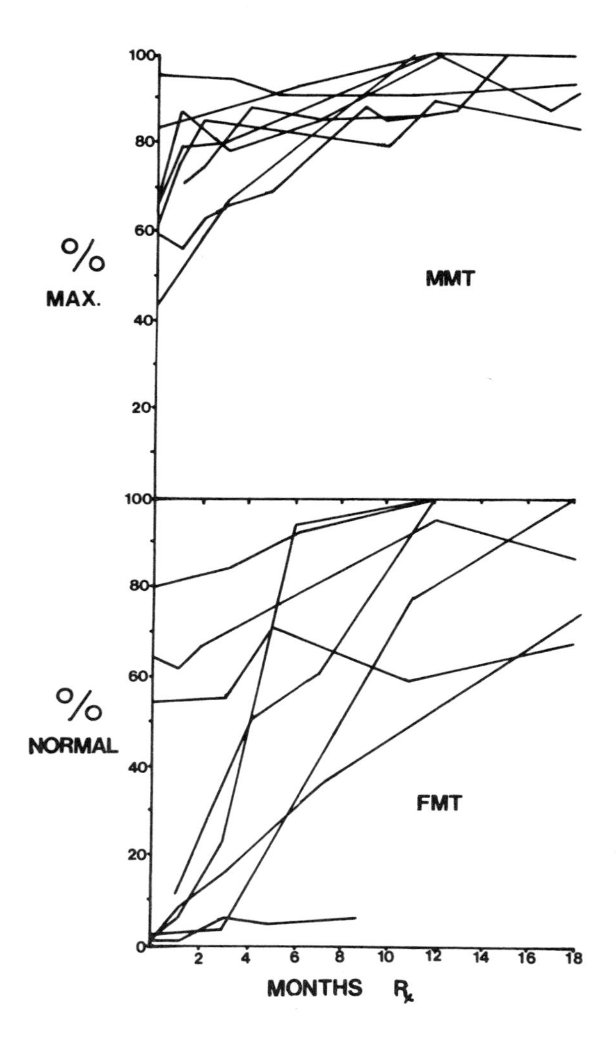

FIG. 7-2. Manual and functional muscle strength testing results, expressed as % of maximum score and % of scores for age, sex, and size-matched control subjects, respectively, during treatment of polymyositis. MMT improved more quickly than did functional test scores.

conditions. For example, in a recent study(14), changes in static (MMT) and dynamic strength were followed for 1 year in 9 patients during treatment of polymyositis, and were correlated with changes in serum muscle enzymes and histological appearances in serial muscle biopsies. The functional muscle strength tests (FMT) consisted of bicep curls and full-arm abductions using small barbell weights for the upper limbs, and squats for the lower limbs, assuming the patient's body weight to be the load. Patients were asked to perform as many repetitions as possible in 1 min at a steady rate, and the *muscular effort* was calculated as weight lifted (kilograms) x number of repetitions x fractions of 1 min that patient could exercise (kilopond-meter-minute).

For comparison, 30 normal volunteers (20 women and 10 men), matched as far as possible for age and weight with the patients, were also studied and the patients' FMT scores were expressed as a percentage of the scores achieved by the appropriate control group. Figure 7-2 shows the MMT scores expressed as a percentage of the theoretical maximum score possible, at different times during treatment, compared with the dynamic test results. It was evident that the rate of functional improvement was far less rapid than the static strength assessments would suggest, and this seemed to correlate in general terms with the architectural characteristics of the muscle biopsies, which remained abnormal throughout the period of observation, particularly with regard to the persistent excess of small type IIc fibers.

The pathological process in polymyositis is one of patchy muscle fiber destruction accompanied by vigorous regenerative activity, which may ultimately result in complete recovery of muscle function; the observed muscle strength at any time will presumably reflect the balance between these two processes. The fundamental process in ALS, on the other hand, is a progressive decline in the number of upper and lower motor neurons, and secondary neurogenic muscular atrophy. The only readily quantifiable index of that process is measurement of muscle strength. Sobue et al. (15, 16) and Kawamura et al. (17) confirmed earlier observations of a selective loss of large myelinated fibers derived from large α motor neurons in the lateral group nuclei of the anterior horns in ALS, and Sobue's group found a linear relationship between the number of preserved large myelinated fibers in ventral nerve roots and muscle strength, measured using a manual muscle testing system (15). A similar relationship was found between strength and number of intact anterior horn cells, and the extent of loss of neurocytons and large myelinated fibers also increased with disease duration (16). Axonal degeneration was evident at all stages of the disease, but there was no evidence of proximal axonal sprouting, and the authors concluded that distal axonal sprouting and resulting reinnervation and fiber-type grouping had little impact on the relentless march of the disease and progressive decline in strength. It can therefore be reasoned that in ALS, serial measurements of static (isometric) strength *in individual muscle groups* should show a linear decline with time and that a decrease in the rate of decline observed during a trial of therapy might indicate a true biological effect of treatment. Most trial protocols do include observations of this type, but differ in the methods of measurement employed.

MEASUREMENT OF STATIC MUSCLE STRENGTH

Factors Affecting Observed Static Muscle Strength

Several factors determine the reproducibility and reliability of strength measurement data. These can be classified as *intrinsic* or inherent to the muscle or subject under test,and *extrinsic*, pertaining to the measurement system. The strength and endurance of a muscle or muscle group is dependent on its anatomical configuration (fusiform or pennate); the fiber-type profile (proportions of oxidative and glycolytic fibers); and by its vascular supply, although the latter is of relatively little importance in the context of maximal voluntary contraction measurements, during which the blood flow falls to near zero (18).

Intrinsic Factors

The normal fiber-type composition has been determined for most muscles (19), but it is well known that these profiles are not immutable and can be altered by specific training patterns.Aerobic endurance training increases the proportion of type 1(oxidative) fibers, whereas strength and power training using isometric and high-load dynamic techniques increases the proportion and size of type 2 (glycolytic) fibers, with predictable effects on observed static strength measurements(20). For practical purposes, however, the two chief factors determining strength are body size and age (12). In normal young and middle-aged subjects, the strength of a muscle group is directly proportional to its cross-sectional area. Men are generally stronger than women, but this appears to be a reflection of their greater muscle bulk rather than some intrinsic property of male muscle, and a single linear relationship has been shown between isometric strength of the quadriceps and body weight for both men and women (21). Isometric strength declines with age, with maximal strength developing at approximately 30 years of age, decreasing to some 80% of this peak at age 65 in men and 70% in women (12). This decline has been linked to preferential fallout of fast-twitch glycolytic fibers in aging muscle, which results in loss of isometric strength in excess of reduction of muscle bulk (22).

Extrinsic Factors

Finally, all strength measurements rely to a considerable extent on the cooperation and enthusiasm of the subject being tested. It can be shown that in normal individuals the force of a maximal voluntary contraction of the quadriceps is the same as the force elicited by tetanic stimulation of the femoral nerve (21) and,although a poor voluntary effort will obviously produce inac-

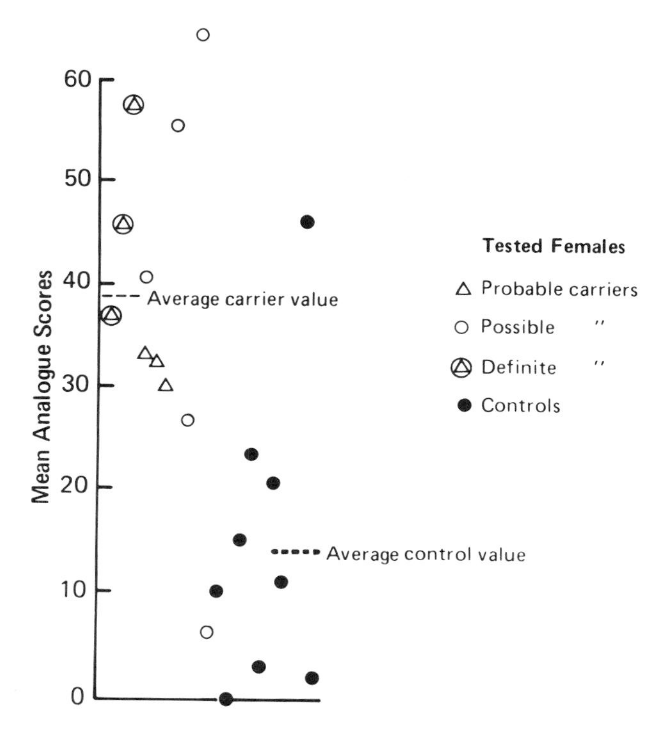

FIG. 7-3. Average analog scores on manual muscle strength testing in 11 Duchenne muscular dystrophy carriers and 9 control subjects. [Reproduced from Lane et al. (28) with permission.]

curate and irreproducible data, it is general experience that patients with organic neuromuscular disorders are cooperative and that measurements on such individuals give acceptable reproducibility. Several factors contribute to the variation observed: the accuracy of the instruments being used, which should be calibrated against known loads; normal fluctuations in strength that occur during the course of the day; and the feedback and rapport between tester and subject. Coefficients of variation (standard deviation/mean x 100) in recent studies of static strength measurements in normal individuals using hand-held dynamometers (3, 23) and the quadriceps testing chair(23) have given values of 5–15%, with test/retest correlations of approximately 0.9, although variation in patients with neuromuscular diseases and significant weakness is usually greater. One recent study found that the subject contributes some 80% of this variance, and the observer only 2–3% but, in another study, variation was significantly less on serial testing by a single experienced observer compared with multiple testers(5). It is clearly desirable that individual laboratories establish their own limits of inter- and intrapersonal variation for the various test systems used.

MANUAL MUSCLE STRENGTH TESTS

Manual muscle strength testing (MMT) remains the most popular method of strength assessment, in view of its convenience and simplicity. The muscle strength grading system originated by Lovett was standardized by Kendall (25), and the principles and definitions were further modified in the United Kingdom by the Medical Research Council scheme (26). For research purposes, gradings are usually converted to integers and are summed to give a strength "score."

MMT can be both sensitive and reproducible in experienced hands.For example, less than 10% of carriers of the Duchenne muscular dystrophy (DMD) gene exhibit weakness on routine clinical examination, but Roses et al. (21) performed careful MMT on 25 known and possible carriers and found significant weakness in all cases, particularly in proximal shoulder and pelvic girdle muscles. In a subsequent blind-controlled study (28), 11 DMD carriers and 9 matched female controls were studied using identical techniques, converting strength gradings to integer analogs. The carriers proved to be significantly weaker than the controls (Fig. 7-3), and, as in the first study, the difference was most marked in certain proximal muscles. The physiotherapists performing the testing were able to correctly distinguish the carriers from controls on this basis in all but three cases. To attempt to eliminate observer bias introduced by the slightly depressed affect of some of the carriers, a subsequent blind-controlled study of 4 previously untested carriers and 7 mothers of children who were inpatients in the pediatric wards was undertaken. The total analog scores in the two groups were similar to the earlier study (Table 7-2), the carriers being significantly weaker; all four carriers were correctly identified by the testers, but there were two "false positives."

Myometry and Strain-Gauge Measurements

MMT are adequate for cross-sectional studies of this type but have two major shortcomings. First, they generate ordinal data,and although the use of integer conversion is reasonable as a first approximation, comparisons of myometry and MMT assessments have shown that the intervals between different grades are not equal; the system is not linear (24). A point of even greater importance in terms of longitudinal studies, such as treatment trials in ALS, is that MMT are inherently insensitive to *changes* in strength, because gradings are confined by specific definitions. A progressive linear decline in strength during an interval will be masked when assessed by MMT, until a change of grade is reached. *Myometry* provides cardinal data, and although the same problems concerning technique pertain as regards interaction of patient and examiner, and the necessary and consistent adoption of optimal positioning for maximal torque, comparative studies have shown that myometry is superior to MMT in

Table 7-2. *Manual Muscle Strength Testing Scores in Single-Blind Study of Duchenne Muscular Dystrophy (DMD) Carriers and Controls*

Subject no.	Analog score	Physiotherapists' prediction	Status[a]
1	35	C	N[b]
2	0	N	N
3	30	C	C
4	0	N	N
5	10	N	N
6	23	C	C
7	27	C	N[b]
8	8	N	N
9	8	N	N
10	19	C	C
11	56	C	C

[a] N denotes normal control; C denotes a DMD carrier.
[b] Incorrectly diagnosed.

terms of sensitivity to minor degrees of weakness and changes in strength (4). Experience with myometry and handgrip strength measurements in ALS in our laboratory are described elsewhere in this volume (Chapter 19).

The use of strain-gauge systems to measure maximal voluntary contraction (MVC) minimizes the problem of observer–subject interaction to some extent. Both MMT and myometry are limited in that the subject's strength is being compared with the observer's own strength. Although this rarely poses problems, these methods are relatively insensitive to changes in large, powerful muscles. Strain-gauge systems such as the quadriceps chair and arm-strength strain gauge are the most direct means of accurate static muscle strength measurement available, but each is dedicated to examination of specific muscle groups. These limitations could be largely overcome by the use of isokinetic dynamometry systems such as Cybex II and Lido, which can be used to measure MVC when used in static mode; their main drawback is their cost.

CONCLUSIONS

Although methods of muscle strength measurement in humans have been described and forms of strength have been defined in terms of their unit dimensions, no one test can adequately describe strength, and tests must be selected in light of their validity to the condition in question, and with regard to sensitivity and reproducibility. It can be argued that serial measurements of static muscle strength (maximal voluntary contraction) reflect the pathogenesis and clinical progression of ALS and should provide a means of detecting a biological response to treatment.

REFERENCES

1. Iddings MD, Smith LK, Spencer WA. Muscle testing. Part 2 (reliability in clinical use). *Phys Ther* 1962;41:249–56.
2. Lillenfeld AM, Jacobs M, Willis M. A study of the reproducibility of muscle testing and certain other aspects of muscle scoring.*Phys Ther Rev.* 1954; 34:279–89.
3. Edwards RHT, Hyde S. Methods of measuring muscle strength and fatigue. *Physiotherapy* 1977; 63:51–5.
4. Wadsworth CT, Krishan R, Sear M, Harrold J, Neilsen DH.Inter-rater reliability of manual muscle testing and hand-held dynametric muscle testing. *Phys Ther* 1987; 67:1342–7.
5. Wiles CM, Karni Y, The measurement of muscle strength in patients with peripheral neuromuscular disorders. *J Neurol Sci* 1983;46:1006–31.
6. Greenwood RJ, Newsom-Davis J, Hughes RAC, et al. Controlled trial of plasma exchange in acute inflammatory polyneuropathy.*Lancet* 1984; 1:877–9.
7. Murray NMF, Wiles CM, Karni Y, Newsom-Davis J. Intensive plasma exchange in acute inflammatory polyneuropathy. *Ann Med Interne(Paris)* 1984; 135:144.
8. Osterman PO, Lundemo G, Pirsaken R, Fagius J, Philstedt P, Siden A, Safwenberg J. Beneficial effects of plasma exchange in acute inflammatory polyradiculoneuropathy. *Lancet* 1984;2:1296–8.
9. Raphael JC, Chastang C. Cooperative French Group: cooperative randomised trial of plasma exchange (PE) in Guillain-Barré syndrome (GBS). Preliminary results. *Ann Med Interne(Paris)* 1984; 135:32.
10. McKann G. Plasmapheresis and acute Guillain-Barré syndrome.*Neurology* 1985; 35:1046–1104.
11. Färrkilä M, Kinnunen E, Haapenen E, Ilvanainen M. Guillain-Barré syndrome: quantitative measurement of plasma exchange therapy.*Neurology* 1987; 37:837–40.
12. Asmussen E. Muscle strength. *Scand J Clin Lab Invest* 1969;110(Supp):106–8.
13. Moffroid M, Whipple R, Hofkosh J, Lowman E, Thistle H. A study of isokinetic exercise. *Phys Ther* 1970; 49:735–46.
14. Lane RJM, Emslie-Smith A, Mosquera IE, Hudgson P. Clinical,biochemical and histological responses to treatment in polymyositis. *J R Soc Med* 1989: 82; 333–8.
15. Sobue G, Matsuoka Y, Mukai E, Takayanagi T, Sobue I. Pathology of myelinated fibres in cervical and lumbar ventral spinal roots in amyotrophic lateral sclerosis. *J Neurol Sci* 1981;50:413–21.
16. Sobue G, Sahashi K, Takahashi A, Matsuoka Y, Muroga T, Sobue I.Degenerating compartment and functioning compartment of motor neurones in ALS: possible process of motor neurone loss. *Neurology* 1983; 33:654–7.
17. Kawamura Y, Dyck PJ, Shimono M, Okazaki H, Tateishi J, Doi H. Morphometric comparison of the vulnerability of peripheral motor and sensory neurones in amyotrophic lateral sclerosis. *J Neuropathol Exp Neurol* 1981; 40:667–75.
18. Humphreys PW, Lind AR: The blood flow through active and inactive muscles of the forearm during sustained hand-grip contractions. *J Physiol (Lond)* 1963; 166:120–35.

19. Johnson MA, Polgar J, Weightman D, Appleton D. Data on the fibre types in thirty-six human muscles. An autopsy study. *J Neurol Sci* 1973; 18:111–29.
20. Kakkinen K, Alen M, Komi PV. Changes in isometric force and relaxation time, electromyographic and muscle fibre characteristics of human skeletal muscle during strength training and de-training. *Acta Physiol Scand* 1985; 125: 573–85.
21. Edwards RHT, Young A, Hosking GP, Jones DA. Human skeletal muscle function: description of tests and normal values. *Clin Sci Mol Med* 1977; 52:283–90.
22. Anianson A, Hedberg M, Henning G-B, Grimby G. Muscle morphology,enzyme activity and muscle strength in elderly men: a follow-up study. *Muscle Nerve* 1986; 9:585–91.
23. Scott OM, Hyde SA, Goddard C, Dubowitz V. Quantitation of muscle function in children: a prospective study in Duchenne muscular dystrophy. *Muscle Nerve* 1982; 5:291–301.
24. Van der Ploeg RJO, Oosterhuis HJGH, Reeuvekamp J. Measuring muscle strength. *J Neurol* 1984; 231:200–3.
25. Kendall HO, Kendall FP, Wadsworth GE. *Muscles: testing and function* (2nd ed.). Baltimore: Williams and Wilkins; 1971.
26. *Aids to the examination of the nervous system.* London:Balliere Tindall, 1986.
27. Roses MS, Nicholson MT, Kircher CS, Roses AD. Evaluation and detection of Duchenne's and Becker's muscular dystrophy carriers by manual muscle testing. *Neurology* 1977; 27:20–5.
28. Lane RJM, Maskrey P, Nicholson GA, et al. An evaluation of some carrier detection techniques in Duchenne muscular dystrophy. *J Neurol Sci* 1979; 43:377–94.

Amyotrophic Lateral Sclerosis,
edited by F. Clifford Rose.
Demos Publications, New York © 1990.

Therapeutic Trials in Amyotrophic Lateral Sclerosis: Measurement of Clinical Deficit

Theodore L. Munsat, Patricia Andres, and Linda Skerry

Neuromuscular Research Unit and MDA/ALS Treatment and Research Center, Tufts-New England Medical Center, Boston, Massachusetts, U.S.A.

It is a fair observation that neurology, as a medical discipline,is regarded as a specialty less concerned with therapeutics than with lesion localization and accurate diagnosis. This legacy from the founders of our specialty has left us relatively naive in clinical trial design. For example, compared with our colleagues in oncology and infectious disease, we lack tradition and experience in sophisticated trial design, quantitative measurement techniques, and statistical analysis. There are few among us who can be easily identified as resource specialists in clinical trials.

The view has been expressed that sophisticated trial design is not actually necessary for neurologic diseases and that all we really need to do is to listen carefully to the individual patient and that when an effective treatment becomes available it will be clear to all. This view holds that expensive and time-consuming trials are not really needed. This is a peculiar perspective, a residual of the neurologist's basic therapeutic nihilism, and is contrary to the perspective of patients with these diseases and contrary to recent experience in other fields of medicine. This view does great disservice to patients and their families, who perceive the disease from a different yet equally valid perspective and who believe that any amount of drug benefit is meaningful. This view also fails to appreciate the history of cancer chemotherapy in which substantive disease arrest was the result of many trials of therapeutic agents that initially produced only modest benefit.

We would therefore propose that neurologists engage in a major effort to develop those skills and techniques necessary to carry out meaningful and cost-effective therapeutic trials. There is great need, in our judgment, for neurologists to develop the experience and resources to be in a stronger position to make meaningful progress in therapeutic intervention.

Therapeutic trials in amyotrophic lateral sclerosis and related diseases have suffered from defective design as much as trials for any other neurologic disease have — maybe even more so.Only recently have attempts been made to construct trials that meet the rigid criteria of sound trial design (1,2). This chapter is concerned with certain aspects of trial design in ALS, particularly the development of measurement techniques.

DISEASE SPECIFICITY

For a measurement system and protocol to be effective, it must be disease specific. Although the same neurologic examination is used to diagnose stroke and ALS, an evaluation system used to detect the effects of a therapeutic intervention or to define the natural history of a disease must be designed specifically for that disease. Clinical neurologic deficit in ALS is confined to the voluntary motor system and is limited to a combination of upper motor neuron (UMN) and lower motor neuron (LMN) deficit.This makes the task of ALS protocol design relatively simple, at least more so than for stroke and multiple sclerosis, which may involve sensory and cognitive as well as motor deficit. The ALS trial design task, then, is to devise a measurement system that is sensitive to small changes within the voluntary motor system.

INCLUSION CRITERIA

It is essential to assure homogeneity of the patient population under study. It is especially important to do so in view of increasing evidence that the clinical features of ALS may result from diverse causes. Strict definitions of the disease must be adopted early in the design process. It is preferable to exclude all atypical cases from study. Rather, the total sample size should be reduced, if necessary, because the inclusion of only a few inappropriate patients could seriously influence the outcome of the study.

ALS, in common with other degenerative neurologic diseases, has no specific biochemical marker. Diagnosis is made through clinical examination and laboratory testing. Clinical and laboratory criteria for the diagnosis should include positive features as well as certain exclusions. Although it is usually easy for the experienced clinician to diagnose ALS, ensuring the purity of the sample selected for a clinical trial demands special care. Any atypical patient should be excluded, including ALS patients with significant sensory complaints or deficit, and those with dementia.

Patients with significant cervical spondylosis without bulbar involvement pose a particular problem. These patients should also be excluded, even if progression of UMN and LMN deficit follows successful surgical decompression. Until further data suggest otherwise, patients with familial ALS should be excluded or evaluated separately.

Patients whose ALS is associated with plasma-cell dyscrasia (3) should certainly be excluded, because some of these patients have been shown to respond to immunotherapy, which is not true of patients without serum protein abnormalities.

In our view, only patients with both clinical UMN and LMN deficit should be included in trials. Clearly, occasional patients with ALS may present with only UMN deficit. In these patients, electrophysiologic studies or muscle biopsy will often provide the necessary evidence of denervation. A similar, and somewhat more difficult to establish situation, is the presence of UMN signs in patients presenting with mainly LMN deficit. Whether a particular degree of reflex hyperactivity or spread is pathologic or not becomes a clinical "judgment call." In this regard, it is important to note that in ALS, positive Babinski responses are uncommon (10% in our experience). When strongly positive Babinskis are present, cervical spondylosis or a demyelinating disorder should be considered.

Certain published studies have included patients with only LMN or only UMN deficit. Patients with only LMN deficit have a much more favorable outlook and are indistinguishable from those with late-onset spinal muscular atrophy. Patients with only UMN deficit probably have a demyelinating disorder, as recent evidence — especially with the advent of magnetic resonance imaging — suggests (4).

Our inclusion criteria for admission to a drug study are based on a narrow definition of the disease, which includes the following elements: (a) a combination of both UMN and LMN deficit at multiple levels; (b) evidence of progression, (c) an absence of neurologic involvement outside the voluntary motor system; (d) no evidence of a primary disease that could cause the deficit, particularly cervical spondylosis or plasma cell dyscrasia.; (e) a patient early enough in the process to be able to complete the study; (f) a patient with a good understanding of his/her disease and the goals of the study; (g) an informed and supportive family; and (h) a patient who can engage in the project without serious financial hardship.

EXCLUSION CRITERIA

The major exclusion criteria are the converse of the above. In addition, we exclude women of childbearing age who do not practice adequate contraception and patients with uncompensated medical illness of any type.

MEASURING STRENGTH

An effective clinical trial cannot be carried out without a reliable and valid measurement instrument and without knowledge of the natural history of the disease under study. The latter depends on the former. The terms "reliable" and "valid" have a special statistical meaning in the context of trial design."Reliable" refers to test reproducibility over time for the same examiner (intrarater reliability) or for different examiners(inter-rater reliability). Reliability variance has a direct impact on sample size, i.e., the wider the variance on test–retest, the larger the number of patients required to achieve statistical significance.

"Validity" is a term used to designate the accuracy and sensitivity with which the function in question is being measured. In ALS, we are interested in measuring the extent of damage to the voluntary motor system. Expressed in another way,"validity" asks the question, Does the measurement instrument actually measure what we want to measure and what we think we are measuring? For example, a rating scale that assesses impairment in climbing stairs might be measuring a change in joint function or pulmonary capacity and not the voluntary motor system.

The issue of validity is intimately related to the experimental hypothesis of the study. Thus, if one asks the question, "Does drug X stop or slow the loss of motor neurons?" then a testing instrument should be used that measures, as directly as possible, motor neurons. On the other hand, if the question asked is, Does drug X result in improved function of the patient regardless of the mechanism by which this improvement occurs? then it might be appropriate to use a rating scale.

Practical considerations must be resolved early. They include the time involved in testing individual patients (many of whom will be significantly disabled), patients comfort and safety, and of course the financial cost and personnel required to carry out the study successfully.

MEASURING UMN DEFICIT

ALS is a unique disease in which clinical deficit is confined to the voluntary motor system. It is characterized by a combination of UMN and LMN loss, and the relationship between the two is unclear. Evidence suggests that the UMN damage is not the cause of the LMN loss or the reverse. Our natural history data (5) suggests that UMN and LMN loss proceed at a similar rate in the same region of the body, implying that the injurious process is damaging the voluntary motor system in its entirety. However,this conclusion must remain speculative until we have a more direct (valid) way of measuring UMN deficit. The inability to measure UMN deficit reliably is a serious problem, not only in ALS but also in clinical studies of other diseases. There is in fact no direct, accepted way to measure UMN deficit. Current physiologic techniques that attempt to do so are relatively crude, lack reproducibility, vary greatly with the baseline status of the patient, and require expensive and time-consuming technology. Physiologic procedures that purport to measure the conduction of central pyramidal pathways have been introduced and are discussed elsewhere. They use electrical and, more recently, magnetic stimulation and are potentially very useful — but will require more study. In the meantime, it will be necessary to use less direct techniques, such as repetitive movement measurement or clinical rating scales. This remains a serious and important challenge for the future.

MEASURING MOTOR UNIT FUNCTION

Accurately measuring the number of functioning motor neurons or motor units is at the heart of the issue of ALS clinical trial design. A number of physiologic techniques for counting motor units are available (6), most of which are based on the technique originally reported by McComas (7). These techniques still have major limitations, including a seriously undesirable overlap of normal and pathologic values and a restriction to the testing of only a small number of muscle groups.

Biochemical assays of blood or urine, and whole-body muscle mass measurements assess only muscle bulk and are not only very indirect ways of measuring motor units, but also are subject to change with alterations in the patient's eating habits and nutritional state.

Imaging techniques have been used successfully by some to measure muscle bulk and at times can be helpful in establishing a diagnosis, but this approach also lacks specificity and validity and is more appropriate for studying primary muscle disease than disease characterized by denervation and reinnervation.

Because the most characteristic and measurable clinical defect in ALS is strength loss, we believe that the primary measurement technique in ALS trials should be the measurement of strength. Strength measurement is currently the most direct manifestation of motor neuron loss. Although marked UMN loss can also result in strength reduction, the amount of strength loss due to UMN deficit in most ALS patients at any stage of their disease would appear to be small. Measurement of force assesses the net loss of strength due to both UMN and LMN loss.

Traditionally, strength is measured by Medical Research Council grading of the manual muscle test (MMT). As we have pointed out previously (2), the MMT technique has grave deficiencies. Although reliability is high, this high reliability is achieved at the expense of a pronounced loss of sensitivity, particularly at the stronger end of the scale. The grades of good and normal (4 and 5) may reflect as much as 97% of the patient's muscle strength. MMT produces ordinal data, i.e., data that are not uniformly incremental (interval).

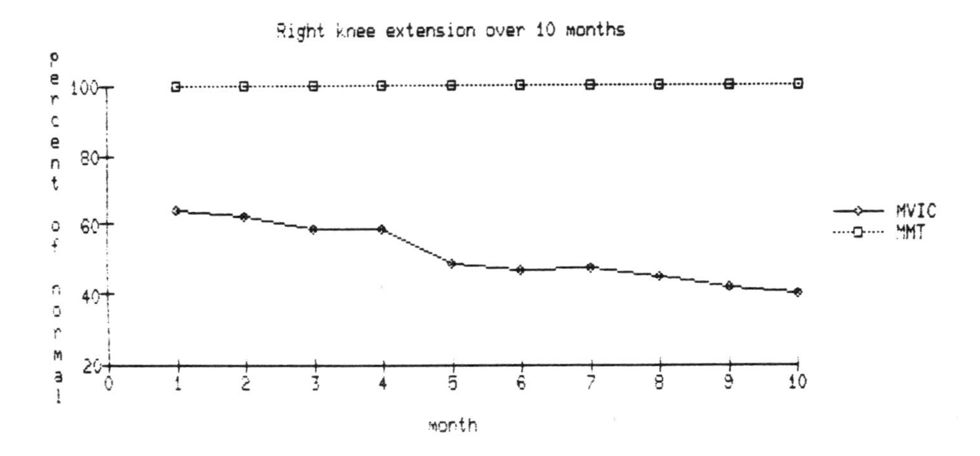

FIG. 8-1. Strength of the right quadriceps muscle of a patient with ALS is measured using manual muscle testing (MMT) and maximal voluntary isometric contraction (MVIC) during a 10-month period. Note that MMT indicates that strength remains at 100% while MVIC declines from 64% to 40% of normal during the 10-month period.

Thus, MMT properly uses only nonparametric and statistically less powerful statistical analytic techniques. MMT can miss distinct and substantial loss of strength (motor units) (Fig. 8-1). Although it is the most commonly used technique in ALS trials and is the heart of most ALS testing scales (1,8,9), we would propose that MMT not be used for any drug trial designed to measure reduction in the loss of voluntary motor function.

Few studies have used a measurement instrument based solely on strength measurement. Most have incorporated MMT into a protocol that also uses functional rating scales. Rating scales have been designed to evaluate both historical and observational data. The latter are more reliable. Rating scales have the advantage of being quick, cost effective, reproducible, and can be performed by a relatively untrained observer. However, they also have reduced sensitivity (Fig. 8-2), especially at the upper ranges of strength, where a drug is most likely to be effective. In addition, rating scales produce ordinal data of varying units and when combined with MMT must be subjected to arbitrary statistical conversion. Lastly, because rated performance is such an indirect measure of motor unit function, it is influenced by many extraneous factors including the patient's motivation, general health and nutrition, cardiovascular and pulmonary impairment,and the adequacy of any assistive devices.

Timed functional tasks add an element of objectivity and produce ordinal data. In addition, certain timed functional activities,especially repetitive tapping tasks, provide an estimate of UMN deficit. However, timed functional

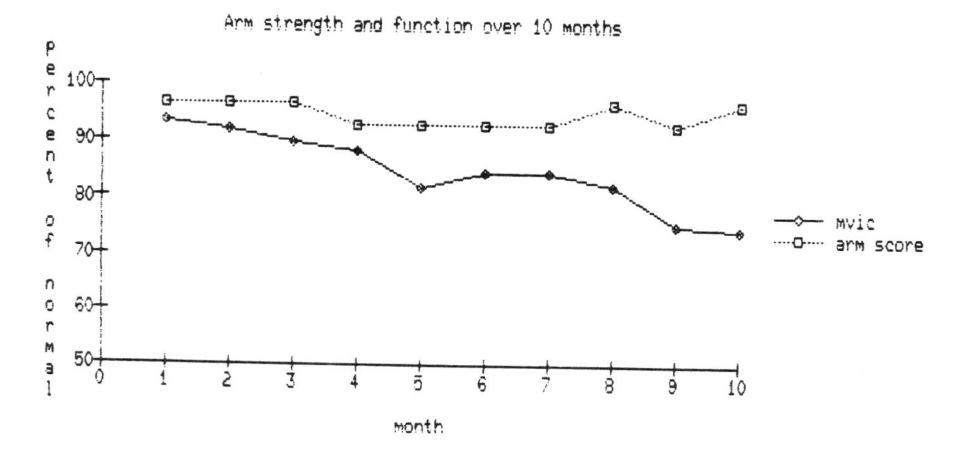

FIG. 8-2. Strength measured using maximal voluntary isometric contraction (MVIC) and a functional rating scale were used simultaneously to measure disease progression during 10 months in a patient with ALS. The rating scale indicated no change while MVIC demonstrates a 20% loss of strength in a linear fashion during this time.

activities often depend on a critical number of motor units and can show a rather dramatic drop off even when the disease process is progressing in a linear manner (Fig. 8-3). Nonetheless, limited timed functional tasks are incorporated into our testing procedure, which we call the Tufts Quantitative Neuromuscular Examination (TQNE) (2).

Several techniques are available for measuring clinical strength. Isotonic strength can be measured using variable resistance devices such as the Cybex. These devices require a major initial expense and can measure only a small number of muscle groups.

Hand-held dynamometers have the advantage of modest cost and portability and provide reproducible interval data. However, they have some of the same shortcomings as MMT. This approach measures strength by "breaking" a posture held and sustained by the patient. It is very insensitive to early loss and in part reflects the strength of the examiner.

In our work we prefer to measure strength by assessing maximum voluntary isometric contraction (MVIC) using an adapted examination table and strain gauge (Fig. 8-4). Force is measured in predetermined standard positions by a trained evaluator. The testing equipment costs less than $3,000. An evaluator can be trained and his or her technique can be validated in 3 days. An average total evaluation of a single patient takes 45 min.

MVIC has several major advantages over other strength-measuring procedures. Intra- and inter-rater reliability is high (2), almost any muscle group is

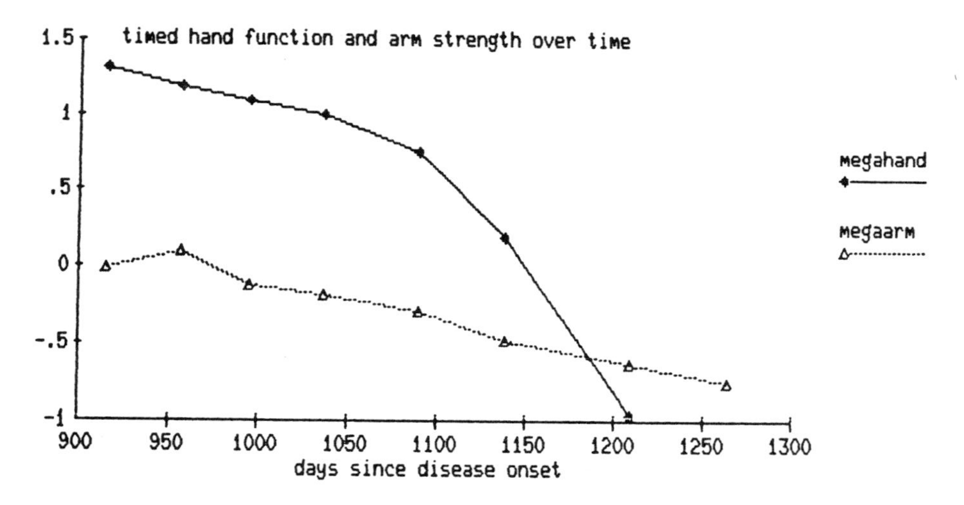

FIG. 8-3. In this patient with ALS there is a continuous linear decline in arm strength while timed hand function drops off sharply after approximately day 1,100.

accessible to testing, the data generated are interval, and the validity of the procedure is high.

STATISTICAL CONSIDERATIONS

During our early work with measurement techniques in ALS, it became clear that the raw data derived from individual measurements required transformation, both to assure equal weighting of test items of inherently different magnitudes and to provide a means of converting different measurement units to a unitary system. Although other statistical techniques are available, we elected to use a "Z" transformation (10,11) based on a reference group of 150 ALS patients. This, on the one hand, allows appropriate representation for muscles both large and small, and on the other, provides comparable results from such functions as pulmonary capacity and strength, and even from timed functional activities.

After Z-converting our data, we analyzed them by a rotated factor analysis. Much to our surprise (and delight) the commonality that resulted had surprising anatomical relevance (Table 8-1). Thus, for example, the strength of the arm flexors was more like that of the extensors than any of the leg muscle groups. We found that individual muscle groups were more like their anatomical neighbors than muscles at a distance were. This quite unexpected result suggests that ALS is a remarkably regional disease and that degeneration of different levels of the neuraxis has different characteristics.

We next decided to use regional composite scores as the basic technique to

Table 8-1. *Extracted Data from a Six-Factor Solution Rotated Factor Analysis of 47 Data Items (Only Values Greater than 0.5 Are Included)*

	Rotated factor loadings (pattern)			
	Factor 1	Factor 2	Factor 3	Factor 4
FVC		0.732		
MVV		0.712		
pa				-0.899
pata				-0.919
phoneR			0.689	
phoneL			0.539	
pegbdR			0.734	
pegbdL			0.501	
shdflexR		0.798		
shdflexL		0.867		
shdextR		0.798		
shdextL		0.878		
elbflexR		0.626		
elbflexL		0.808		
elbextR		0.713		
elbextL		0.820		
gripR		0.598		
gripL		0.615		
hipextR	0.570			
hipextL	0.552			
hipflexR	0.546			
hipflexL	0.608			
kneextR	0.588			
kneextL	0.623			
kneflexR	0.665			
kneflexL	0.750			
dorsiflexR	0.721			
dorsiflexL	0.781			

Reproduced from Andres et al. (10) with permission.

analyze disease. Several features favor using composite scores instead of individual data items. Contrary to what intuitive reasoning might suggest, the use of composite scores actually enhanced the statistical validity of the study. It provides repeated measurement of similar items (as determined by our factor analysis studies) and also cancels out positive and negative errors in the measurement system. More important, because both our factor analysis and our natural history studies strongly suggest that ALS is a very regional disease

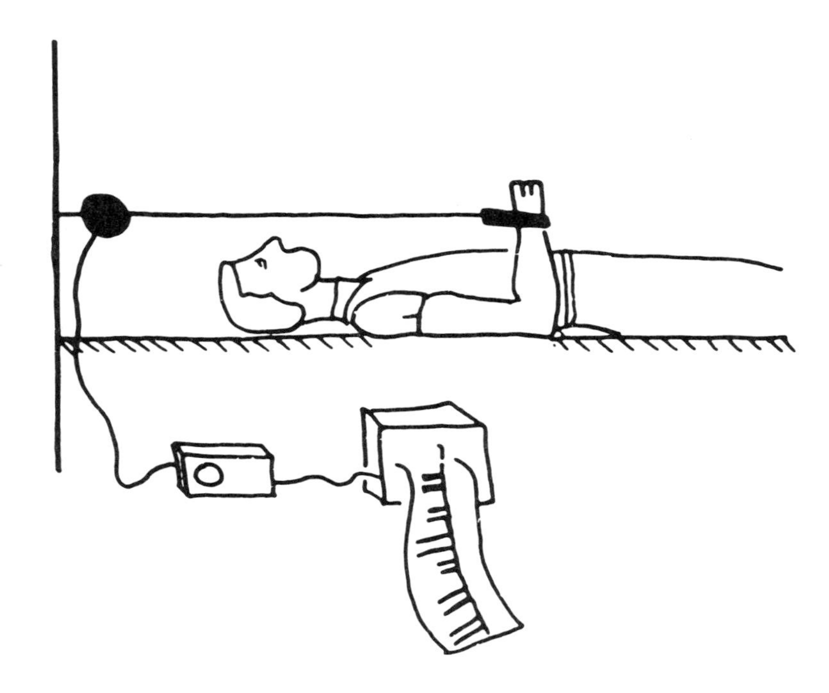

FIG. 8-4. Maximal isometric voluntary contraction (MVIC) is performed on a standard examination table with aluminum uprights and adjustable rings. A nylon strap is positioned on the limb.The strap is connected to the strain gauge, which is attached to a ring on an immobile upright. The strap and strain gauge remain parallel with the table. Force is transduced by the amount of distortion within the strain gauge, and then is amplified and recorded on a strip-chart recorder.

and that the time of disease onset and rates of deterioration have regional characteristics, we believe that the course of ALS should be analyzed regionally to fully understand the meaning of change— either in a natural history study or in a study evaluating therapeutic intervention. Scores that summate function beyond a single anatomical level or summate all functions of a patient can seriously misrepresent the course of the disease. One region in that patient may be progressing quite rapidly while the other may be deteriorating slowly or not at all.

NATURAL HISTORY OF ALS

After constructing and validating our measurement system, we proceeded to study the natural history of the disease. We selected patients for our natural history studies most carefully and excluded any patient who did not fulfill strict criteria for the diagnosis (see "Inclusion Criteria" and "Exclusion Criteria" sections). We then performed TQNEs on each of 50 patients for 8 or more months, analyzing rates and patterns of deterioration. Our results demonstrated that once deterioration begins, it proceeds in a surprisingly linear manner. Deterioration rates among patients varied as much as 20-fold, but deterioration rates between different anatomic areas of the same patient varied less. Deterioration rates were not seriously affected by the patient's sex, age, or the region of disease onset.

We are currently analyzing these data to devise a technique for accurately predicting the future course of deterioration for a particular patient when he or she is first seen. These data should also be useful for designing more efficient and effective clinical trials. We are pleased that other research groups have incorporated this methodology in their study of the natural history of ALS and the effects of therapeutic intervention (12).

THE FUTURE

Those involved with clinical trials in ALS currently find themselves in a unique situation. For the first time in the history of the disease, new hypotheses of etiology and pathogenesis point to a large number of drugs that are candidates for clinical trials. The present challenge is somehow to rank these agents in terms of priority and then to allocate resources to test them in a timely and cost-effective manner. This endeavor requires a coordinated, collaborative clinical research effort similar to that used in cancer therapy trials and the recent Collaborative Investigation of Duchenne Dystrophy supported by the Muscular Dystrophy Association.

Acknowledgment: This study was supported by National Institutes of Health grants MO1RR00054 and RO1NS24623 and by grants from the Muscular Dystrophy Association.

REFERENCES

1. Appel V, Stewart SS, Smith G, Appel SH. A rating scale for amyotrophic lateral sclerosis: description and preliminary experience. *Ann Neurol* 1987; 22:328–33.
2. Andres PL, Hedlund W, Finison L, Conlon T, Felmus M, Munsat TL. Quantitative motor assessment in amyotrophic lateral sclerosis. *Neurology* 1986; 36:937–41.
3. Shy ME, Rowland LP, Smith T, Trojaborg W, Latov N, Sherman W, Pesce MA, Lovelace RE. Motor neuron disease and plasma cell dyscrasia. *Neurology* 1986; 36:1429–36.
4. Miska RM, Pojuna W, McQuillen MP. Cranial magnetic resonance imaging in the evaluation of myelopathy of undermined etiology. *Neurology* 1987; 37:840–3.

5. Munsat TL, Andres PL, Finison L, Conlon T, Thibodeau L. The natural history of motorneuron loss in ALS. *Neurology* 1988;38:409–13
6. Brown WF, Strong MJ, Snow R. Methods for estimating numbers of motor units in biceps-brachialis muscles and losses of motor units with aging. *Muscle Nerve* 1988; 11:423–32.
7. McComas AL. *Neuromuscular function and disorders.* London:Butterworths, 1977.
8. Norris FH, Calanchini PR, Fallat RJ, Panchari S, Jewett B. The administration of guanidine in amyotrophic lateral sclerosis. *Neurology* 1974; 24:721–8.
9. Olarte, MR. Therapeutic trials in amyotrophic lateral sclerosis.In: Rowland LP, ed. *Human motor neuron diseases. Advances in neurology; vol. 36. New York: Raven Press 1982; 555–8.*
10. Andres PL, Finison L, Conlon T, Thibideau L, Munsat TL. Use of composite scores (megascores) to measure deficit in ALS. *Neurology* 1988; 38:405–8.
11. Rosner B. *Fundamentals of biostatistics.* Boston: Duxbury,1982.
12. Festoff BW, Smith RA, Melmed S, Frane J, Sherman B, Finson R, Andres P, Munsat TL. Tufts Quantitative Neuromuscular Exam (TQNE) and amyotrophic lateral sclerosis (ALS) trials in the recombinant age. *Ann Neurol* 1988; 24:138–9.

Amyotrophic Lateral Sclerosis,
edited by F. Clifford Rose.
Demos Publications, New York © 1990.

9

Clinical Appraisal of Progression of Amyotrophic Lateral Sclerosis: A Japanese ALS Scale

Masao Honda

Yokohama City Hospitals, Yokohama, Japan

Japan is no different from other countries in that no amyotrophic lateral sclerosis (ALS) scale has been widely used. I have tried to produce a scale and with trial and error have developed one that I have found satisfactory and herein present.

DESCRIPTION OF THE SCALE

The scale is of the ordinal type, with a maximum upper value of 500 and a minimum lower value of 0. It evaluates 77 items, more numerous than those ordinarily included in scales of this type. Table 9-1 and 9-2 show what these 77 items are, and in Table 9-3 the recording paper for this scale is shown in which each item is described briefly with the maximum points for the item. A relatively larger number of check items and more points are allotted in this scale to those parts of the body related to finer and more sophisticated motor functions. This is because a larger number of motor neurons are involved in these functions and motor disabilities in these parts indicate loss of a relatively larger number of neurons. In actually applying this scale to ALS patients, examiners need to follow the instruction book to check the 77 items; to rank the severity of each item, and to decide how many to give to each rank. Most of the motor activities are ranked according to six degrees of severity—normal, minimally impaired, mildly impaired, moderately impaired, severly impaired, totally impaired. Each rank is given a score of 0–5 points. In deciding the severity of motor disability, skill in performing that particular action is taken into consideration together with muscle strength. In a disease such as ALS in which not only the lower motor neurons but also upper motor neurons are involved, this is important

Table 9-1. *Number of Items Evaluated by the Scale According to Different Modes of Evaluation*

Mode	Items
Activity tests	35
Inspection and palpatation of muscles	20
Reflex tests	13
Self-reported activities	7
Muscle tone tests	2
Total	77

because the action may not be well done due to mass movement or spasticity. The activity tests are so devised so that most can be done while the patient remains in the same position, that is, supine.

Muscle atrophy is rated into three ranks: normal, atrophy, and marked atrophy, with a score of 0–2 points. Presence or absence of fasciculation is not taken into consideration in this scale because it is difficult to know clearly what this sign signifies, e.g., it may signify a regenerative or degenerative process. The stretch reflex is checked in seven different tendons on each side: the gag reflex, abdominal reflex, Babinski's reflex, Rossolimo's reflex and Hoffman's reflex and ankle clonus each constitutes a check item, the presence of which is given a score of 2 at the maximum. Self-reported activities, which include speaking, swallowing, changing and buttoning clothes, feeding, breathing, and walking are graded into 4–6 ranks with a maximal score of 4–10 points. Muscle tone is evaluated by passive movement of extremities and a score of 0 is given for normal, 2 for increased or reduced tone, and 4 for markedly increased or reduced tone. Paralysis of respiratory muscles is evaluated by the ratio of minimum over maximum chest circumference; a ratio > 1.04 is normal with a score of 0; those between 1.04 and 1.02 and between 1.01 and 1.0 are given scores of 4 and 8, respectively. The ratio of 1 means no movement of the chest cage and is given a score of 10 points. Grip strength is measured by hand

Table 9-2. *Number of Items Evaluated by the Scale According to Different Parts of the Body*

Body part	Items
Facial, oral, and bulbar	13
Upper extremities	26
Trunk	16
Lower extremities	22
Total	77

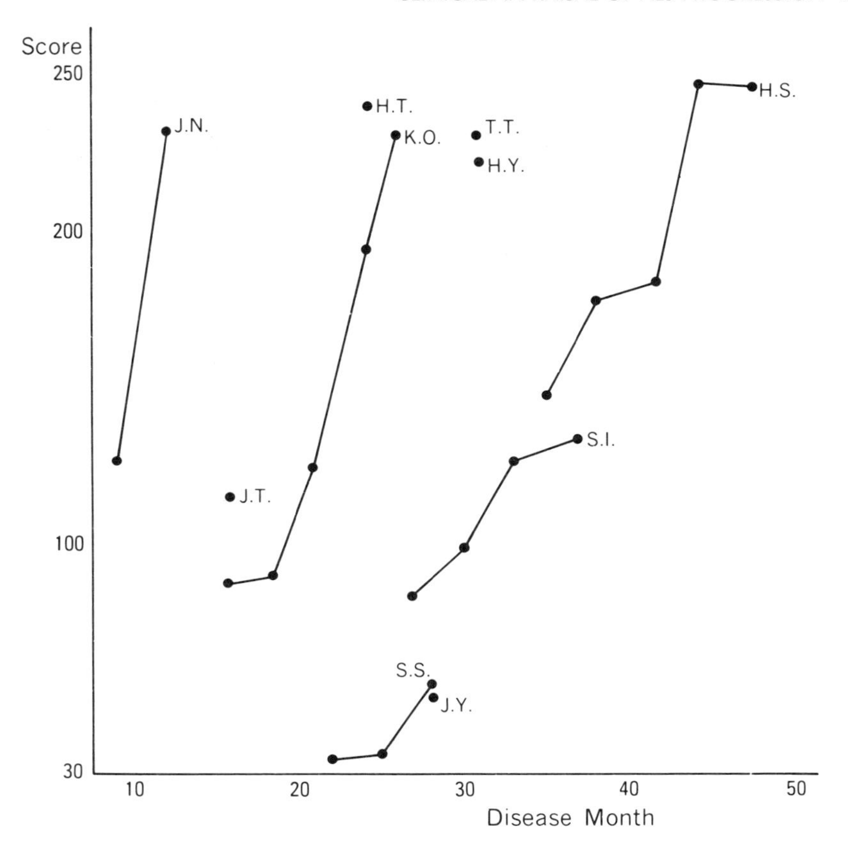

FIG. 9-1. The total ALS scores are recorded for 10 different patients monitored during 9–47 months.

dynamometer and strength > than 20 is scored as 0. Strength between 10 and 20 and below 10 are given scores of 1 and 2, respectively. When the patient cannot hold a dynamometer, the score is 3.

RESULTS

Figure 9-1 shows the total ALS scores as a function of disease month for 10 patients. Table 9-4 shows the correlation between total scores and ALS clinical stages described in a previous report (1). Those patients who were in the initial stage and who could still live productively had an average score of 44, whereas those in the early advanced stage who were still ambulatory had an average score of 139. In the late advanced stage, when the patients were bedridden, the

Table 9-3. *Recording Paper for the Scale Showing Items Evaluated and Maximum Points for Each*

No.	Item	Points	Side
1.	Clench teeth	(3)	R L
2.	Masseter	(2)	R L
3.	Jaw jerk	(2)	R L
4.	Move eyebrow	(5)	R L
5.	Close eye	(5)	R L
6.	Open mouth	(5)	
7.	Close mouth	(5)	
8.	Snout reflex	(2)	R L
9.	Obricularis oris	(2)	
10.	Swallow	(10)	
11.	Speak	(10)	
12.	Gag Reflex	(2)	
13.	Tongue	(10)	
14.	Bend neck	(5)	
15.	Extend neck	(5)	
16.	Shrug shoulder	(5)	R L
17.	Raise arm	(5)	R L
18.	Deltoid	(2)	R L
19.	Change clothes	(5)	
20.	Adduct arm	(5)	R L
21.	Pectoralis major	(2)	R L
22.	Bend Elbow	(5)	R L
23.	Biceps	(2)	R L
24.	Extend elbow	(5)	R L
25.	Triceps	(2)	R L
26.	Bend wrist	(5)	R L
27.	Wrist flexors	(2)	R L
28.	Extend wrist	(5)	R L
29.	Wrist extensors	(2)	R L
30.	Adduct fingers	(5)	R L
31.	Abduct fingers	(5)	R L
32.	Bend fingers	(5)	R L
33.	Extend fingers	(5)	R L
34.	Feed oneself	(5)	R L
35.	Button	(5)	
36.	Thenar	(2)	R L
37.	Hypothenar	(2)	R L
38.	Grip	(3)	R L
39.	Biceps jerk	(2)	R L
40.	Triceps jerk	(2)	R L
41.	Brachioradialis jerk	(2)	R L
42.	Hoffman reflex	(2)	R L
43.	Muscle tone in upper ext.	(4)	R L
44.	Breath	(10)	
45.	Move chest	(10)	
46.	Intercostalis	(2)	R L
47.	Rectus abdominis	(10)	
48.	Abdominal reflex	(1)	R L
49.	Turn on bed	(5)	R L
50.	Scapular winging	(2)	R L
51.	Upper erector spinae	(2)	R L
52.	Lower erector spinae	(2)	R L
53.	Gluteus	(2)	R L
54.	Hamstrings	(2)	R L
55.	Raise hips	(6)	
56.	Bend hip	(5)	R L
57.	Extend hip	(5)	R L
58.	Abduct hip	(5)	R L
59.	Adduct hip	(5)	R L
60.	Bend knee	(5)	R L
61.	Extend knee	(5)	R L
62.	Quadriceps	(2)	R L
63.	Extend foot	(5)	R L
64.	Gastrocnemius	(2)	R L
65.	Dorsiflex foot	(5)	R L
66.	Tibialis anterior	(2)	R L
67.	Muscle of sole	(2)	R L
68.	Knee jerk	(2)	R L
69.	Ankle jerk	(2)	R L
70.	Babinski's reflex	(2)	R L
71.	Rossolimo's reflex	(2)	R L
72.	Ankle clonus	(2)	R L
73.	Muscle tone in lower ext.	(4)	R L
74.	Sit on bed	(10)	
75.	Stand	(4)	
76.	Get up	(2)	
77.	Walk	(4)	

Name: Date: Total score: R, right side; L, left side.

Table 9-4. *Independent Clinical Stage and ALS Scores*

Clinical stage	No. of observations	Average ALS score
Initial	4	44
Early advanced	13	139
Late advanced	4	207
Terminal	3	264

average score was 207, and in the terminal stage, when the patient had respiratory distress of more than moderate degree, the average score was 264.

DISCUSSION

The course of ALS is variable because the disease progresses rapidly in some patients and only very slowly in others. It is important, therefore, to study what produces this difference because it may be possible to find a clue to a therapy. The rate of progression of ALS has often been discussed in relation to the duration of the illness, but this is not correct because many patients die prematurely due to bulbar paralysis, and short survival may not be the same as rapid progression. The disease may not progress at the same speed during the whole course, so that we need to analyze more closely the mode of progression in individual patients, and for that we need to have a scale by which we can monitor the progression of ALS quantitatively. The ALS score presented here is based on the result of evaluation of 77 items, which include motor function of facial and bulbar muscles as well as that of the muscles of the trunk and extremities. Inclusion of such symptoms as difficulty in closing the eyes, opening the mouth, or turning in bed, which are often omitted by other scales, has made the scale more complete. It may be argued that an excessively large number of items makes the scale difficult to use, but this scale is not time-consuming and does not impose much of a burden on patients because the activity tests are so devised that most of them can be done while the patient remains in the same position, that is, supine. For example, extension of neck or hip is examined with patients in the supine position as a strength with which to resist an attempt to bend them and not as is usually done in the prone position. In advanced stages, when the patient is immobile, this is helpful both to patient and examiner.

One of the features that make this scale distinct from other ALS scales is that it reflects the extent of motor neuron loss rather than how badly the patient is incapacitated. As is well illustrated by the homunculus caricature drawn by Penfield, a relatively larger number of upper motor neurons are involved in the fine and sophisticated movements of the face, tongue, and hand than in crude movements of the trunk and extremities. This is also true with lower motor neurons. Therefore, impairment of the motor functions of these parts of the body indicates loss of larger numbers of neurons than that of the functions of other parts. In this scale, by allotting a larger number of check items and therefore more points to the movement of face, tongue, and hands, the total score is made to represent the extent of motor neuron loss rather than the severity of patients' motor disability.

Another feature of this scale is that the degree of motor dysfunction is not decided by muscle strength alone. In a disease such as ALS, in which both upper and lower motor neurons are involved, the muscle test is not easy to perform and it may not reveal the true nature of the motor disability. Therefore, when necessary, skill in performing the action is evaluated and rated together with muscle strength.

Respiratory function is evaluated by measuring minimal and maximal chest circumferences. This is because ALS patients may become unable to hold the mouthpiece due to paralysis of orbicularis oris in the advanced stage, and evaluation of the function may become impossible or inaccurate if spirometry is used for that. Measurement of chest circumference is easy and this makes scoring possible until the end of the disease.

Our experience with this scale is still limited, but it has clearly shown that the extent of motor neuron loss can be much different even in patients with a similar duration of ALS, and it has also suggested that the rate of progression of the illness may be different in different stages in the same patient.

Although it was designed to reflect neuronal loss, the scale has been shown to correlate with the independent evaluation of clinical stage and can also be considered to indicate to some extent the clinical status of ALS patients.

Thus, the scale will help us to clarify further the course of ALS and, hopefully, the factors that can influence it. It will also serve as an indicator of a patient's clinical status.

REFERENCE

1. Honda M. Clinical strategies in dealing with ALS. In: Tsubaki T, Yase Y, eds. *Amyotrophic lateral sclerosis.* Amsterdam: Elsevier Science, 1988.

Amyotrophic Lateral Sclerosis,
edited by F. Clifford Rose.
Demos Publications, New York © 1990.

10

Charting the Course in Amyotrophic Lateral Sclerosis

Forbes H. Norris

ALS Center, Pacific Presbyterian Medical Center, San Francisco, California, U.S.A.

The need to assess progression in amyotrophic lateral sclerosis (ALS) by scoring each patient at certain times in the illness was apparent in the 1960s as large-scale treatment efforts began. Stimulated by the late Israel Wechsler, Norris and Engel (1) had already tried cancer treatments in selected ALS patients who also had various malignant diseases, and Engel, Norris and others (2,3) were trying programs of nutritional therapy plus certain corticosteroids in other ALS patients. At that time, the need for an unbiased, population-based ALS cohort was not known, and the possibility of favorable placebo responses seemed unlikely.

In multiple (disseminated) sclerosis, Kurtzke (4) had presented a single staging method and Tourtellotte et al. (5) had devised a more complex scoring system. The former seemed too simple or, viewed another way, unlikely to detect small changes, whereas the Tourtellotte system seemed complex and time consuming, perhaps obtaining more data than was really necessary to score the individual patient. A major, continuing problem in ALS is patient fatigue, which seems especially marked when the disease progression is rapid, in addition to the usual problems of patient compliance, ability to travel for examinations, etc.

Simplification of the Tourellotte score, including appropriate modifications for ALS patients (e.g., elimination of the visual fields and acuity) was developed and, with sufficient experience, seemed adequate for scoring ALS.

Table 10-1. *ALS Score for Case NS17 24 Months After Entry*

Item	Weight			
	3 (Normal)	2 (Impaired)	1 (Trace)	0 (No use)
1. Hold up neck	X			
2. Chewing	X			
3. Swallowing	X			
4. Speech	X			
5. Roll over in bed		X		
6. Do a sit-up			X	
7. Bowel-bladder pressure	X			
8. Breathing	X			
9. Coughing		X		
10. Write name			X	
11. Work buttons, zippers			X	
12. Feed self		X		
13. Grip/lift self			X	
14. Grip/lift book/tray			X	
15. Grip/lift fork/pencil		X		
16. Change position		X		
17. Climb stairs —1 flight				X
18. Walk — 1 block				X
19. Walk — 1 room		X		
20. Walk — assisted	X			
21. Stand up from chair			X	
22. Change position	X	X		
		Hyper/hypo	Absent	Clonic
23. Stretch reflexes —arms		X		
24. Stretch reflexes —legs		X		
	Absent	Present	Hyperactive	Clonic
25. Jaw jerk	X			
	Flexor	Mute	Equivocal	Extensor
26. Plantar response —right				X
27. Plantar response —left	X			
	None/rare	Slight	Moderate	Severe
28. Fasciculation				X
29. Atrophy —face, tongue	X			
30. Atrophy —arms, shoulders				
31. Atrophy—legs, hips		X		X
32. Labile emotions	X			
		0 to Mild		Moderate to severe
33. Fatigability	—		—	X
34. Leg rigidity	—		—	X
Patient total 59 =	33	+20	+6	+0
Normal total 100 =	96	+ 4	+0	+0

METHODS

This "ALS score" was published in brief in 1974 (6). Major revisions were made in 1982, but only minor alterations were made subsequently. An actual ALS score from a recent patient is presented in Table 10-1, and this and other scores from the same patient are shown in Fig. 10-1. The Appendix gives more details.

RESULTS AND DISCUSSION

It will be apparent immediately to any experienced neurologist that this scoring system contains several subjective or "soft" items, specifically items 2, 7, 12, and possibly 32 (ALS is a depressing disease). Fasciculation (item 28) varies from day to day in most patients. Fatigue (item 33) nearly always increases during the evaluation and in the presence of depression. Figure 10-1 shows the total ALS scores in each evaluation plus a subtotal derived by subtracting the scores for these "soft" items. The graphs reveal the same rate of deterioration.

One advantage of such a Tourtellotte-type system is that particular items can be emphasized or not, depending on the analysis, e.g., data on the plantar

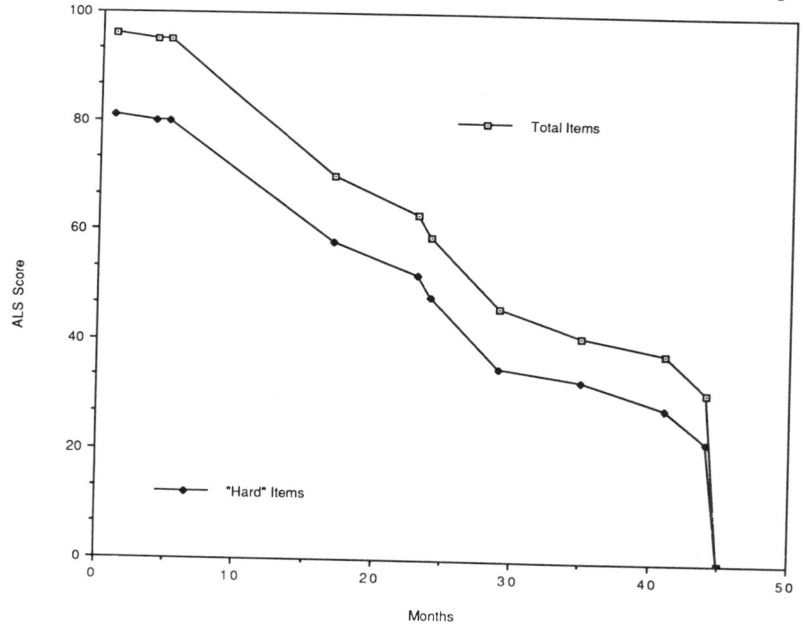

FIG. 10-1. The ALS scores in patient NS17 during 45 mo from May 1983 to January 1987, when death occurred. The total score (top curve) is paralleled by a subtotal of "hard scores" (see text). The 24-mo score is detailed in Table 10-1. This patient was also presented as case 1 in Norris and Fallat (8).

Table 10-2. *ALS Scores by Two Neurologists in Evaluation of 11 Patients Who All Deteriorated During the Study Period*

Patient no.	Scores by neurologist 1			Scores by neurologist 3		
	Entry	At 3 mo	6 mo	Entry	At 3 mo	6 mo
1	82	80	72	79	69	70
2	77	68	66	75	70	61
3	56	68[a]	66[b]	67	74[a]	67[b]
4	80	81	77	88	81	78
5	39	39	43[b]	41	39	31
6	74	64	57	78	56	58[a]
7	84	82	74	79	81[a]	62
8	76	66	37	63	51	34
9	89	86	79	85	85	78
10	81	84[a]	79	—	78	71
11	62	66[a]	24	64	50	—

[a] ALS scores improved in 2-test comparisons.
[b] Deterioration during 6 mo not indicated by ALS scores.

response is easy to retrieve. Another advantage is simplicity. Unless the evaluation is interrupted, e.g., by uncontrollable emotional lability, the follow-up scores can be done in approximately 10 min after the patient is undressed. As a practical matter, I often watch the patient in the final acts of undressing and moving to the examination table and, later, moving off the examination table and beginning to dress, which provides essential data without need for formal testing. The initial evaluation, when we do not yet know one another, usually requires approximately 30 min, and of course the sympathetic attention to new or other problems (e.g., the residual swelling from a recent ankle sprain) nearly always lengthens the follow-ups, but the ALS score is usually made easily and quickly. The only equipment required is a reflex hammer and a score sheet. Scoring can be done as easily during a house call, so follow-ups are readily obtained.

A major concern in any scoring system is reproducibility. Figure 10-1 suggests, because we all know that the course in ALS is usually downhill, that this ALS score is generally reproducible, and therefore valid for charting the course. Table 10-2 shows the scores in 11 patients studied independently and blindly by two neurologists in an assessment of octacosanol (3,7). In this study, each patient was considered clinically to have deteriorated at least slightly between each evaluation at entry, 3, and 6 months. The asterisks in Table 10-2 mark the evaluations in which the ALS scores not only failed to show the disease progression but actually indicated slight improvement, and in one case both examiners' scores failed to show the deterioration after 6 months. This experience suggests that the ALS score can mislead in approximately 8% of the two-test comparisons and in 3% of three-test comparisons. We have no com-

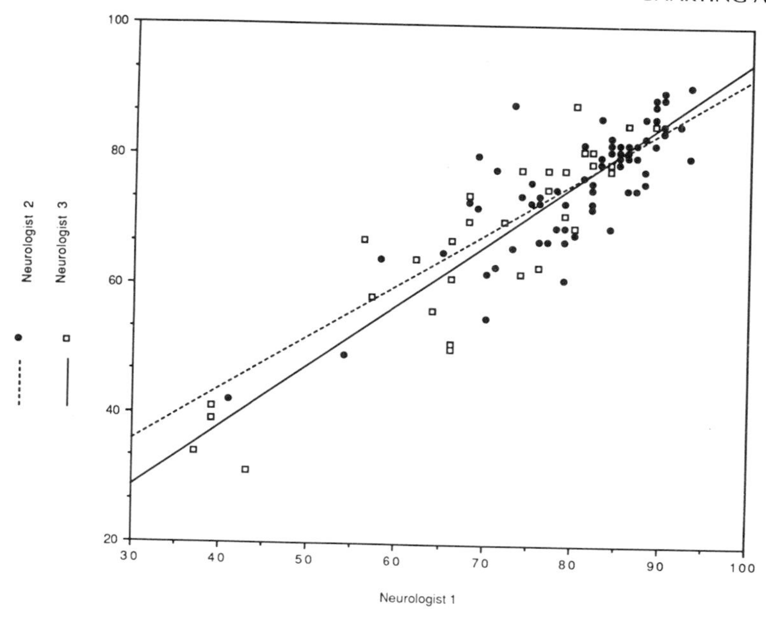

FIG. 10-2. Comparison of scores made independently and recorded blindly by neurologist 1 (horizontal) with neurologists 2 and 3 (vertical). The correlation coefficients are 0.81 and 0.90, respectively.

parable data on the much smaller number of ALS patients experiencing transient improvement.

Another estimate of reliability is provided by comparing the scores of different neurologists. We have done this formally (and blindly) on two different occasions (3,6,7) with results presented in Fig. 10-2. In all of these evaluations, the individual scores were collected separately by a third party and were stored until the conclusion of each study. As reported earlier, the scores of neurologist 2 and myself had a correlation coefficient (*R*) of 0.81 (6). The *R* for neurologist 3 and myself was 0.90.

In many respects, these *R* and the lack of absolute clinical correlation (Table 10-2) indicate a troublesome level of reliability, particularly for the detection of small clinical alterations. We recognized this early on and in 1974, Dr. Kwei Sang Ü and I devoted the better part of a year to improving the ALS score, without success. Such improvements as counting pins transferred per minute from table to cup, counting finger taps per minute, etc. (5) all succumbed to patient cooperation–fatigue factors.

Meanwhile, collaborating physical and respiratory therapists were enrolled to carry out independent (and blind) assessments as reported elsewhere (6). We continue to emphasize an independent pulmonary evaluation (8) but have omitted the physical therapy measurements for several reasons, mainly the problem of maintaining the therapists' interest in the face of the usual ALS deterioration plus declining financial support for our work, and patient fatigue in an additional 30–60 min of testing.

The pulmonary function tests are most important in the ALS patient, especially when early breathing–coughing muscle impairment develops, so recently we have reported a staging method for such involvement (8). Meanwhile, returning to a point made earlier regarding the Kurtzke stages (4) of multiple (disseminated) sclerosis, it seems that the reliability–reproducibility of this ALS score may barely discriminate changes in ALS better than the Kurtzke-type stages, so it is of great interest to hear about the simple ALS staging method developed by Hillel and associates (9 and chapter 11). There are also several other scoring or staging methods developed to detect slight alterations in the course of ALS (10,11). In recommending any of these to colleagues, the important considerations are the goal of the scoring system (e.g., small versus large changes), its simplicity/complexity, and acceptability by patients.

CONCLUSIONS

Charting the clinical course in ALS became important with the development of large-scale clinical trials at multiple centers from the mid-1960s. The evaluations described for multiple (disseminated) sclerosis by Kurtzke and Tourtellotte led to development of an "ALS score" at the ALS Center in San Francisco. Combined with special pulmonary muscle evaluations, always carried out blindly in a separate department, this ALS score has been used continuously since a major modification in 1972. Its main advantages are simplicity for the examiner and for the patient, and ease of cooperation without much fatigue. In follow-up evaluations, the testing is usually completed within 10 min by an experienced neurologist. Some of the items in the score are subjective, historical, or variable, but deletion of these items does not greatly change the clinical profile given by the scoring system. Two other neurologists, after < 1 h of instruction, obtained correlation coefficients with the author of 0.81 and 0.90. In up to 8% of two-evaluation comparisons by the same examiner, the score may falsely indicate improvement when clinical worsening has actually occurred, but in three-evaluation comparisons this error falls to approximately 3%. The simplicity of this ALS score must be emphasized when considering more elaborate (also more expensive, complicated, fatiguing) scoring systems.

Acknowledgment: The early phases of this work were supported by the John A. Hartford Foundation. The octacosanol study was supported by the Shelly Byers Chapter of the ALS and Neuromuscular Research Foundation, San Francisco. The current review is also supported by the ALS and Neuromuscular Research Foundation. Dr. P. R. Calanchini has given generous support and collaboration during the past 20 years, Dr. E. H. Denys for 13 years. Leben Harmon gave assistance with the statistics, and Vicki Tiernan did the layout and typing.

APPENDIX

Explanation of ALS Score Presented in Table 10-1 and Figure 10-1

ITEM DESCRIPTION	SCORE
1. Hold up head(test)—No problem	3
Droops when tired, or unable to complete chin–test	2
Always droops without support collar, only clears pillow supine	1
Cannot clear pillow when supine	0
2. Chewing (history)—No problem	3
Requires some soft or blenderized foods, some rest periods	2
Completely soft/blenderized diet, frequent rest periods	1
Food must be pushed to back of mouth	0
3. Swallowing (test)—No problem drinking a glass of water	3
Aspirates some water but not saliva during entire examination	2
Aspirates saliva occasionally, drools frequently	1
Water runs out of mouth, aspirates saliva frequently	0
4. Speech (test)—Normal throughout visit	3
Any problem during visit	2
Barely understandable simple phrases	1
Grunts, groans, rare intelligible sounds	0
5. Roll over (test)—Turn readily to at least one side from supine on examination table	3
Any problem (may be due to severe arm weakness but score here also)	2
Barely turns with great effort to just one side	1
Needs assistance to turn	0
6. Sit up (test)—Sit to full vertical from supine on examination table	3
Clears head, shoulders but not trunk without pulling	2
Clears head but not shoulders without pull/lift	1
Requires lift of both head, trunk	0
7. Bowel/bladder pressure (history)—No apparent problem	3
Problem bearing down; needs laxative or stool softener every week	2
Needs laxative or softener more often, occasional enema	1
Enema needed more often than not	0
8. Breathing (test)—No problem during entire visit	3
Dyspnea arriving at office or during strength testing	2
Dyspnea in ordinary conversation	1
Respiratory distress	0
9. Cough (test)—Examiner unable to restrain lower chest in coughing (hold from behind)	3
Cough effective but examiner able to restrain chest	2
Cough usually ineffective, e.g., multiple shallow coughs after aspiration	1
Cough ineffective	0
10. Write (test)—Write name, address; spouse confirms normalcy	3
Any legibility problem with name, address	2
Unable to complete name, address, or mainly illegible	1
Only able to make marks	0
11. Buttons, zippers (test)—Buttons shirt; may use both hands, time not limited but no assist devices; pull zipper closed	3

Unable to complete above without aid	2
Only able to do two buttons with assist devices, half of zipper	1
Unable to perform above, near-full assistance needed	0
Feeding (history) No problem or needs simple assist devices only, e.g., large handles	3
Requires help cutting meat or needs more assist devices, e.g., finger splints, arm slings/pivots, etc.	2
Unable to cut or fork but can raise food to mouth	1
Must be fed	0
13. Grip/lift self(test)—Pulls self erect from supine position with one hand	3
Above with great effort or both grips necessary	2
Above using trunk flexors (examiner palpates abdomen)	1
Requires lift or pull by examiner	0
14. Grip/lift book, tray(test)—Lifts large book from lap to face level	3
Clears lap but cannot lift to face	2
Lifts pocket book from lap to face	1
Clears lap with pocket book but cannot lift to face	0
15. Grip/lift fork, pencil (test)—Holds pencil to write, legibility not considered	3
Lifts pencil but unable to grip enough to mark	2
Lifts pencil clear of table only briefly	1
May move pencil but cannot lift clear	0
16. Change arm position (test)—Lift both arms over head from lap	3
Arms clear lap but not shoulders	2
Moves both arms from lap to arm rests	1
Wiggles arms but not enough to move from lap	0
17. Climb stairs (test)—Climbs one flight without pausing or pulling	3
Climbs one flight but resting or pulling on rail required	2
Climbs two or more steps unaided	1
Climbs less than two steps, probably needs lift onto examination table	0
18. Walk (test)—Walks one block (office corridor four times without pause, may wear favorable shoes, ankle brace, etc., < 5 min	3
Completes the distance with problems of any type or needs > 5 min	2
Completes only with assist or multiple rests	1
Cannot complete	0
19. Walk one room (test 15 ft)—Completes without difficulty	3
Any problem	2
Completes but needs minimal assist or is exhausted	1
Cannot complete without substantial aid including cane/crutch	0
20. Walk assisted (test only if assist required above, score three if item 19 scores one or better)—Completes one room using cane/crutch or holding examiner arm	3
Cannot complete without other assistance	2
Takes steps in transfer from chair to examination table	1
Legs drag in assisted transfer	0
21. Stand (test)—Stands readily from standard chair, no pushing	3
Any problem	2
Actively assists but needs lift to complete rise	1
Needs lifting throughout	0

22. Change leg position (test)—Raises each leg to 45° in supine position 3
    Clears table but one leg cannot reach 45° 2
    Only clears table briefly, or one leg completely paralyzed 1
    Only ineffective wiggles 0
23. Biceps, brachioradialis, triceps muscle stretch reflexes (test)—All within the broad range of normal and symmetrical 3
    Asymmetry or at least one clearly abnormal 2
    Any three absent, the remaining three only trace responses 1
    Any three clonic 0
24. Quadriceps, Achilles, internal hamstring muscle stretch reflexes (test)—as in item 23
25. Jaw jerk (test)—Self-explanatory
26, 27. Plantar responses (test)—Non-reactive includes response failure from toe extensor paralysis. Babinski's "sign of the toe" only is evaluated; ignore fanning, do not perform the other "confirmatory" tests.
28. Fasciculation (observe throughout examination, patient stripped to standard underwear, no T-shirt)— No neuromuscular drugs, e.g., pyridostigmine, during the previous 24 h
29–31. Wasting (atrophy) (observe)—Self-explanatory
32. Labile emotions (history and observation)—No problem, spouse confirms 3
    Occasional inappropriate weeping or giggling 2
    At least daily lability 1
    Weeping (rarely laughter) with most stimuli, e.g., entering office 0
33. Fatigabilitiy (test)—No abnormality ranging to occasional reduction in strength during examination with rapid recovery in minutes 2
    Frequent reduction in strength during examination or general decline in function with time 0
34. Leg rigidity (test)—Muscle tone normal or slightly increased in both legs, or normal in one but moderate (resists gravity) in the other; no muscle relaxant in 24 h 2
    Moderate rigidity in both, or board-like in one, or worse 0

REFERENCES

1. Norris FH, Engel WK: Carcinomatous amyotrophic lateral sclerosis. In: Brain R, Norris FH, eds: *The remote effects of cancer on the nervous system.* New York and London: Grune & Stratton, 1965:24–34.
2. Engel WK, Hogenhuis LAH, Collis WJ, et al. Metabolic studies and therapeutic trials in amyotrophic lateral sclerosis. In: Norris FH, Kurland LT, eds. *Motor neuron diseases.* New York and London: Grune & Stratton, 1969:199–208.
3. Norris FH, Denys EH. Nutritional supplements in amyotrophic lateral sclerosis. In: Cosi V, Kato AC, Parlette W, Pinelli P, eds. *Amotrophic lateral sclerosis.* London: Plenum, 1987:183–9.
4. Kurtzke JF. Further notes on disability evaluation in multiple sclerosis, with scale modifications. *Neurology* 1965;15:654–61.
5. Tourtellotte WW, Haerer AF, Simpson JF, Kuzma JW, Sikorsky J. Quantitative clinical neurological testing. I. *Ann NY Acad Sci* 1965;122:480–505.

6. Norris FH, Calanchini PR, Fallat RJ, Panchari S, Jewett B. The administration of guanidine in amyotrophic lateral sclerosis. *Neurology* 1974;24:721–8.
7. Norris FH, Denys EH, Fallat RJ. Trial of octacosanol in amyotrophic lateral sclerosis. *Neurology* 1986;36:1263–4.
8. Norris FH, Fallat RJ. Staging respiratory failure in ALS. In: Tsubaki T, Yase Y, eds. *Amyotrophic lateral sclerosis: recent advances in research and treatment.* Amsterdam: Excerpta Medica, 1988:217–22.
9. Hillel AD, Miller RM, McDonald E, Konikow N, Norris FH. ALS severity scale. In: Tsubaki T, Yase Y, eds. *Amyotrophic lateral sclerosis: recent advances in research and treatment.* Amsterdam: Excerpta Medica, 1988:247–52.
10. Andres PL, Hedlund W, Finison L, et al. Quantitative motor assesment in amyotrophic lateral sclerosis. *Neurology* 1986;36:937–41.
11. Appel V, Stewart SS, Smith G, Appel SH. A rating scale for amyotrophic lateral sclerosis: description and preliminary experience. *Ann Neurol* 1987;22:328–33.

Amyotrophic Lateral Sclerosis,
edited by F. Clifford Rose.
Demos Publications, New York © 1990.

11

Amyotrophic Lateral Sclerosis Severity Scale

Allen D. Hillel, Robert M. Miller, Kathryn Yorkston, Evelyn McDonald, Forbes H. Norris, and Nancy Konikow

Veterans Administration Medical Center and University of Washington, Seattle, Washington, U.S.A.

Amyotrophic Lateral Sclerosis Severity Scale (ALSSS) is a staging system designed to rate the functional impairment of an ALS patient. The scale designates a numerical level of function in each of five areas so that objective data regarding a patient's clinical condition can be reported. The five areas are (a) speech, (b) swallowing, (c) lower extremity function, (d) upper extremity function, and (e) vital capacity.

The intent of the severity scale is to provide a degree of objectivity for (a) evaluation of disease progression, (b) designating disease levels for which specific treatment guidelines can be recommended, and (c) staging patients for inclusion in treatment trials.

METHODS

Each of the five sections of the severity scale is based on the progressive decline of function in one specific area: speech—intelligibility of verbal communication; swallowing—chewing and swallowing function; lower extremity function—use of the lower extremities for walking; upper extremity function—use of the upper extremities for dressing and hygiene (Tables 11-1–4); and vital capacity—vital capacity as measured on a hand-held respirometer.

Table 11-1. *Speech*

Rating	Description
Normal speech processes	
10: Normal speech	Patient denies any difficulty speaking. Examination demonstrates no abnormality.
9: Nominal speech abnormalities	Only the patient or spouse notices speech has changed. Maintains normal rate and volume.
Detectable speech disturbance	
8: Perceived speech changes	Speech changes are noted by others, especially during fatigue or stress. Rate of speech remains essentially normal.
7: Obvious speech abnormalities	Speech is consistently impaired. Affected are rate, articulation, and resonance. Remains easily understood.
Intelligible with repeating	
6: Repeats message on occasion	Rate is much slower. Repeats specific words in adverse listening situations. Does not limit complexity or length of messages.
5: Frequent repeating required	Speech is slow and labored. Extensive repetition or a "translator" is commonly used. Patient probably limits the complexity or length of messages.
Speech combined with nonvocal communication	
4: Speech plus nonverbal communication	Speech is used in response to questions. Intelligibility problems *need* to be resolved by writing or a spokesperson.
3: Limits speech to one-word responses	Vocalizes one-word responses beyond yes/no; otherwise writes or uses spokesperson. Initiates communication nonvocally.
Loss of useful speech	
2: Vocalizes for emotional expression	Uses vocal inflection to express emotion, affirmation, and negation.
1: Nonvocal	Vocalization is effortful, limited in duration, and rarely attempted. May vocalize for crying or pain.
X Tracheostomy	

Each of the first four scales provides 10 rating choices (1–10). The examiner should acquire information for rating by taking a history from the patient and from a limited physical examination. In addition, information gathered from family members is not only allowed but encouraged. In some cases, the examiner will have to estimate what a patient *can* do or *should* do (i.e., needs). For example, if the patient claims to be walking without assistance (a rating of 7 or higher), but admits to having fallen on a number of occasions, the patient

Table 11-2. *Swallowing*

Normal eating habits	
10: Normal swallowing	Patient denies any difficulty in chewing or swallowing. Examination demonstrates no abnormality.
9: Nominal abnormality	Only patient notices slight indicators such as food lodging in the recesses of the mouth or sticking in the throat.
Early eating problems	
8: Minor swallowing problems	Complains of some swallowing difficulties. Maintains essentially a regular diet. Isolated choking episodes.
7: Prolonged time/smaller bite size	Meal time has insignificantly increased and smaller bite sizes are necessary. Must concentrate on swallowing thin liquids.
Dietary consistency changes	
6: Soft diet	Diet is limited primarily to soft foods. Requires some special meal preparation.
5: Liquified diet	P.O. intake adequate. Nutrition limited to primarily liquified diet. Adequate thin liquid intake usually a problem. May force self to eat.
Needs tube feeding	
4: Supplemental tube feedings	P.O. intake alone no longer adequate. Patient uses or NEEDS a tube to supplement intake. Patient continues to take significant (> 50%) nutrition p.o.
3: Tube feeding with occasional p.o. nutrition	Primary nutrition and hydration accomplished by tube. Receives < 50% nutrition p.o.
NPO	
2: Secretions managed with aspirator and/or medications	Cannot safely manage any p.o. intake. Secretions managed with aspirator and/or medications. Swallows reflexively.
1: Aspiration of secretions	Secretions cannot be managed noninvasively. Rarely swallows.

should be rated as requiring assistance (a rating of 6 or less).

When rating a patient, use the major headings first. Once the appropriate major heading has been chosen, choose one of the two minor headings. The text should be considered as a general description of the minor heading and single specific items of the text should not cause a rating shift. In each case, when choosing a major or minor heading, look at one heading below your choice before settling on a final rating. If you cannot decide between two choices, even after examining the text supplements, choose the less severe (higher number) rating.

Table 11-3. *Lower Extremities (Walking)*

Normal	
10: Normal ambulation	Patient denies any weakness or fatigue. Examination detects no abnormality.
9: Fatigue suspected	Patient suspects weakness or fatigue in lower extremities during exertion.
Early ambulation difficulties	
8: Difficulty with uneven terrain	Difficulty and fatigue when walking long distances, climbing stairs, and walking over uneven ground (even thick carpet).
7: Observed changes in gait	Noticeable changes in gait. Pulls on railings when climbing stairs. May use leg brace.
Walks with assistance	
6: Walks with mechanical device	Needs or uses cane, walker, or assistant to walk. Probably uses wheelchair away from home.
5: Walks with mechanical device *and* assistant	Does not attempt to walk without attendant. Ambulation limited to < 50 ft. Avoids stairs.
Functional movement only	
4: Able to support weight	At best, can shuffle a few steps with the help of an attendant in transfers.
3: Purposeful leg movements	Moves legs purposely to maintain mobility in bed.
No purposeful leg movement	
2: Minimal movement	Minimal movement of one or both legs. Cannot reposition legs independently.
1: Paralysis	Flaccid paralysis. Cannot move lower extremities (except, perhaps, to close inspection).

It is recommended that the examiner use the rating instructions openly in front of the patient and refer to the text to ask the necessarily specific questions. It is also recommended that the examiner rate each patient in the following order: speech, swallowing, lower extremity, upper extremity, and vital capacity.

Vital capacity is measured by using a hand-held respirometer. The patient's nose should be sealed either by a clip or by the examiner's fingers. In some cases, due to lip weakness, the examiner or an assistant might need to help the patient achieve a seal around the respirometer mouthpiece. The use of mask respirometers is discouraged because they are less accurate, especially at low volumes.

The ALSSS takes 5–10 min to administer and provides a means to rapidly

Table 11-4 *Upper Extremities (Dressing & Hygiene)*

Rating	Description
Normal function	
10: Normal Function	Patient denies any weakness or unusual fatigue of upper extremities. Examination demonstrates no abnormality.
9: Suspected fatigue	Patient suspects fatigue in upper extremities during exertion. Cannot sustain work for as long as normal. Atrophy not evident on examination.
Independent and complete self-care	
8: Slow self-care	Dressing and hygiene performed more slowly than usual.
7: Effortful self-care performance	Requires significantly more time (usually double or more) and effort to accomplish self-care. Weakness is apparent on examination.
Intermittent assistance	
6: Mostly independent	Handles most aspects of dressing and hygiene tasks alone. Adapts by resting, modifying (electric shaver), or avoiding some tasks. Requires assistance for fine motor tasks, e.g., buttons, ties, etc.
5: Partial independence	Handles some aspects of dressing and hygiene alone. However, routinely requires assistance for many tasks such as make-up, combing, shaving, etc.
Needs attendant for self-care	
4: Attendant assists patient	Attendant must be present for dressing and hygiene. Patient performs the majority of each task with the assistance of the attendant.
3: Patient assists attendant	The attendant directs the patient for almost all tasks. The patient moves in a purposeful manner to assist the attendant. Does not initiate self-care.
Total dependence	
2: Minimal movement	Minimal movement of one or both arms. Cannot reposition arms.
1: Paralysis	Flaccid paralysis. Unable to move upper extremities (except, perhaps, to close inspection).

evaluate the functional status of an ALS patient. Used serially over a number of visits, the scale can indicate an overall rate of clinical progression of disease, and can act as a guide to determine appropriate supportive treatment.

Acknowledgment: We thank Brenda Townes, Ph.D., Sue A. Wiedenfeld, Ph.D., Clare Maxwell, M.S., Deanna Chew-Friedenberg, Ph.D., Lola Armstrong, and New Road Map Foundation.

Amyotrophic Lateral Sclerosis,
edited by F. Clifford Rose.
Demos Publications, New York © 1990.

12

Bulbar Dysfunction

R. Langton Hewer and P. M. Enderby

Department of Neurology, Frenchay Hospital, University of Bristol, Bristol, England

Dysphagia, choking, dribbling, and dysarthria are among the most distressing symptoms encountered in clinical practice. At any one time, more than 50% of patients with motor neuron disease (MND) will be experiencing these symptoms (1) and the vast majority will do so eventually. The symptoms can be a major cause of social isolation, fear, and depression for both patients and those who care for them.

Despite the obvious importance of bulbar symptoms, there are very few well-validated methods of assessment. As a consequence, many of the techniques used to alleviate bulbar symptoms have not been fully evaluated and their usefulness is in question. The problem is also of importance for those who are evaluating new treatment regimens, such as thyrotrophin stimulating hormone analogs (TSH).

WHY MEASURE?

Measurement of performance is an essential prerequisite for scientific evaluation of all forms of therapy, whether curative or symptomatic (2,3). The availability of standardized measuring techniques of bulbar function would do much to improve the assessment of the many therapies available. Indeed, it is the basis of audit and "good practice" in this important field of medicine. There are three situations in which accurate assessment is required.

1. Curative treatment. Many therapeutic agents are being, or have been, recently evaluated (e.g., TSH). These trials require that bulbar function should be both identified and accurately quantified. Assessment procedures must be reliable and must be capable of identifying at least a 10–15% change in performance.

2. Symptomatic therapy. The value of, for instance, drugs to reduce spasticity of bulbar muscles can best be judged by the standard double blind technique involving the use of a therapy and control group of patients. Again, it is necessary to have tried-and-tested assessment tools.

3. Determining the value of particular therapeutic techniques in individual patients in everyday practice.

WHAT TO MEASURE?

The two main areas that require measurement are, first, the symptoms, e.g., slurred speech and difficulty with swallowing, and second, the anatomical, physiological, psychological, and pathological mechanisms that produce the symptoms.

For example, there may be weakness and/or spasticity of the lips, tongue, palate, and pharyngeal muscles, which fail to act in a coordinated way and that are, in turn, influenced by fear and embarrassment, to produce difficulty with swallowing. Assessment of the end point — swallowing — is clearly important, but it is also essential to identify and quantify the various component factors, which are not the same in all patients. Thus, in some patients, spasticity predominates over weakness and in others the reverse is the case, whereas in others, the two phenomena are balanced. Clearly, the clinical management will depend on the underlying pathological mechanism. If spasticity dominates, it may be appropriate to use anti-spastic drugs and ice. If weakness is the main problem instructional techniques or mechanical support (e.g. a palatal splint) may be required.

The Patient's Symptoms

Table 12-1 lists some of the common bulbar symptoms encountered in MND. In the majority of areas, no well-validated assessment tools exist, but in some cases, they are desperately needed. A particular example is drooling (dribbling), which

Table 12-1. *Some Common Bulbar Symptoms in Motor Neurone Disease*

Dysarthria
Dysphagia
Drooling (Dribbling)
Choking
Blockage of the Nose
Breathlessness
Emotional Lability

Table 12-2. *Underlying Basis of Bulbar Symptoms*

Underlying abnormality	Results
Weakness and/or spasticity of muscles	Many muscles potentially affected, including lips, masseters, tongue, palate, pharynx, vocal chords, neck and respiratory muscles. The results include inability to acquire, chew, manipulate, and swallow food. There may also be impairment of coughing and breathing.
Changes in the amount/consistency of saliva and mucus	These contribute to dribbling, spontaneous choking, and nasal and aural congestion
Dysphagia	This may produce dehydration, weight loss, and exhaustion
Overflow of secretions into trachea	The result is likely to be choking and recurrent respiratory infections
Oral fungal infections	Dysphagia
Emotional/psychological disturbance	Embarrassment, depression, inappropriate laughing/crying, demoralization, and exhaustion. All the above can have a powerful effect on bulbar function.
Respiratory insufficiency	This may produce respiratory distress, impaired cough, and inability to clear the airway

is an unpleasant and humiliating symptom. Identification of the problem is easy, but quantification can be impossible. No method exists for deciding when, for instance, a transtympanic neurectomy should be undertaken.

As already discussed, a wide variety of anatomical, physiological, pathological, and psychological mechanisms may contribute to bulbar symptoms, and Table 12-2 indicates that it is not sufficient simply to assess the patient's symptoms.

HOW TO MEASURE

Assessment involves the identification of lost function (3). Clinical assessment is rarely sufficient and some form of measurement is required that defines the extent and severity of deficits. The following conditions should be fulfilled by any assessment tools used.

1. The technique should be *relevant* to the problem under consideration.
2. The test must be *valid* — i.e., it must measure what it is supposed to measure. For example, if electromyographic (EMG) activity is to be used to

measure spasticity, it must be shown that the test correlates with some clinical measure of spasticity.

3. The test must be both reliable and repeatable. For instance, it must be shown that two or more observers will obtain approximately the same result. Similarly, research assessments must be undertaken by personnel who are neutral and are not involved in the trial. Impartiality is essential. Because most patients tire quickly, there may be marked variations of performance at different times of the day.

4. Sensitivity. The test must be able to detect small changes in the patient's performance, but this sensitivity is usually bought at the cost of reliability, and in practice it is necessary to achieve a balance between these two ideals.

5. Simplicity. Sensitive tests are often complex and time consuming. Ill and anxious patients may not be able to perform reliably, so the twin objectives of sensitivity and simplicity are in conflict. Tests used in everyday clinical situations by busy staff should be simple and quick.

6. Communicability. One of the major merits of assessment procedures is that the results can communicated to others, e.g., most people have an idea of the significance of an IQ of 100. Similarly, a Functional Communication Profile of 70% usually indicates that the patient will be able to communicate quite well in everyday social situations. The great merit of assessment systems involving a numerical score is that the patient's progress can be measured and discussed.

In practice, the number of validated tests used in the assessment of bulbar function is small, but certain tests do exist, and examples of validated and reliable tests are now discussed.

Dysarthria

Dysarthria is one example of a clinical problem that can be assessed with some accuracy. For instance, the Frenchay Dysarthria Assessment (4) involves analysis of various components of speech, including respiration, lips, jaw, palate, laryngeal muscles, tongue, as well as intelligibility. Each item is subdivided into a number of component sections. For example, three components of palatal function are assessed: fluid leakage into the nose, maintenance of position in a resting situation, and function during speech, each being assessed on an 8-point scale with a histogram produced. Such analysis enables the various components of speech in MND to be readily assessed.

Although there are standard tests of intelligibility, for example Tikofsky (1970) (5), and a similar but more objectively standardized test by Yorkston and Beukelman (1980) (6), there are still many problems in accurately gauging the intelligibility of conversation rather than of single words and prescribed sentences. Some with severe dysarthria can still make themselves understood by organizing the context of what they say and exploiting other features, such as facial expression and intonation. Others less severely impaired when analyzing their phonology, may well be less intelligible in conversation, speak too quickly, lack insight, or change the subject too quickly. Thus, intelligibility of single words and sentences does not necessarily correspond with functional intelligibility, and may not be the result of bulbar dysfunction alone.

Dysphagia

Assessment of dysphagia is difficult, and standardized test procedures are not yet in general use. The patient may have difficulty with swallowing food and/or liquids, and this problem may occur at oral or pharyngeal level, frequently at both. The oral phase itself may involve spasticity and/or weakness of the lips, masseters, and/or the tongue, so that there may be problems accepting food into the mouth, with grinding, and/or with propelling the bolus to the back of the throat. The various techniques to assist swallowing can only be effectively deployed if there has been a precise analysis of exactly what has gone wrong.

In the assessment of swallowing, it is important to acquire information about such diverse matters as the length of time required to eat a standard meal, the occurrence and frequency of choking and of nasal regurgitation, as well as hydration and changes in weight.

Despite the evident importance of dysphagia, some reports do not include any detailed analysis of dysphagia and its consequences, and standard tests are not used. For instance, a recent article (7) involving a study of branched-chain amino acids in amyotrophic lateral sclerosis used a 3-point scale to assess the various components of bulbar function: facial movement, tongue movement, palatal movement, dysarthria, and dysphagia. This method of assessment has not been, to our knowledge, validated, and the criteria listed earlier in this chapter are not met. Clearly, there is need for a sensitive and reliable test for dysphagia to be used in clinical trials of drugs as well as in symptomatic management of individual patients. An agent that produces a 20% improvement in function would be regarded as a great advance, so tests that will reliably identify this degree of change are needed.

THE MANAGEMENT OF MND

There are a number of techniques and approaches that, if used intelligently, can do much to avoid the distress of choking, inability to swallow, and dribbling. Norris, et al. (8) summarized the position in 1985 in a particularly valuable article, and it has also been dealt with more recently (9).

Unfortunately, many of the techniques in common use have not been fully evaluated. Their practical usefulness, particularly in situations in which the staff concerned does not have extensive experience, remain in doubt. Table 12-3 lists some of the approaches and techniques frequently used but that await

Table 12-3. *Cricopharyngeal Myotomy — Four Published Studies*

STUDY	MND Only	MND & Other Diagnostic Groups	No. of MND Patients	Deaths Within 2 WK	Results
Mills (10)	—	Yes	17	1 (6%)	6 "Good" 10 "Moderate"
Lebo et al. (11)	Yes	—	38	3 (8%)	24 (64%) Improved 14 (36%) No benefit
Loizou et al. (12)	—	Yes	20	5 (25%)	All Improved
Mady (13)	Yes	—	19	6 (30%)	8 Improved
David (14)	Yes	—	31	6 (19%)	21 (68%) Improved
Totals			106	15 (14%)	64–100% "Improved"

MND, motor neuron disease.

detailed evaluation. Two particular problems have been selected for further brief analysis.

Cricopharyngeal Myotomy (CPM)

Division of the fibers of the cricopharyngeus muscle has been practiced for many years in an attempt to relieve swallowing difficulty, and the technique is recommended in many standard neurological texts.

Preoperatively, it is necessary to undertake a clinical assessment, which should be followed by a barium swallow and video fluoroscopy. Certain preoperative criteria for CPM have been suggested.

Five reports have given details of the results of CPM in 106 patients (Table 12-3) (10–14). The overall postoperative mortality was 14% varying between 6 and 30% in different series. Benefit was reported in 100% of survivors in two studies, and in 64 and 68% in the remaining two studies, but detailed examination of these publications shows that in none was there any attempt to describe the improvement in meaningful terms, such as speed of eating, frequency of choking, or weight gain. Reliance appears to have been placed on clinical impression. Norris et al. (8) report a morbidity and treatment failure rate of less than 5%, but no details were given.

The technique of CPM has not yet been subjected to adequate scientific evaluation, and the number of patients in whom the technique has been used is very small. In virtually none of the studies is there clear-cut evidence of benefit based on the results of objective testing and, overall, the value of the operation is totally unknown. Indeed, discussion at a recent conference on MND elicited the fact that many experienced clinicians have largely abandoned the procedure.

Communication Aids (CAs)

Severe dysarthria can eventually give way to anarthria, and the failure of verbal communication. Some patients remain able to write, at least for a time. Eventually, this too becomes impossible, and some form of communication aid is required. The obvious objective is to enable patients to communicate with their families up to the time of death.

There has been one study of CAs in MND (15), Sixteen patients being assessed with four different aids. Assessment involved, for example, the number of words per minute that could be communicated. The Canon Communicator and Splink were found to be popular with many patients. We are not aware of any other published evaluations of communication aids in MND.

Since 1981 a very large number of CAs have become available. The topic was reviewed recently (16), but not specifically in relation to MND.

Clearly, more studies, using standardized tests of communication, are required if the full potential of communication aids is to be realized. The question as to whether patients, using modern technology, can be enabled to continue communicating with their relatives up to the time of death remains unanswered.

Other areas in which evaluated evidence is lacking include the alleviation of drooling, and the relative merits of nasogastric tubes versus pharyngostomy and gastrostomy.

Other management techniques require evaluation.

1. There is remarkably little information about the opinions and views of patients and those who care for them. Patient satisfaction appears not to be a generally accepted outcome measure, and no techniques to assess it appear to have been published.

2. There is little published information about the terminal few days and actual mode of death in MND. Saunders et al. (17) gave information about 100 cases of MND dealt with in a hospice and this report remains an important and useful contribution, but similar information about patients dying in their own homes is also required, particularly in relation to the amount of terminal distress and fear.

3. There is a remarkable lack of information about what *actually happens* in different parts of the country and world, e.g., it is impossible to ascertain how frequently gastrostomy or pharyngostomy were actually used in the late 1980s. The "success" of the techniques and frequency of complications in unknown.

Table 12-4. *Some Unanswered Questions in the Management of Motor Neuron Disease*

Value of video fluoroscopy in the assessment of dysphagia
The use of drugs — e.g., Mestinon, atropine, and other anticholinergic drugs
The use and indications of surgery to reduce excessive salivation
The indications for nasogastric tube feeding, gastrostomy, and pharyngostomy. What is the safety and acceptability of these procedures?
The indications for cricopharyngeal myotomy, its safety and usefulness
The use of palatal splints to improve the quality of speech an- dease of swallowing
The use of ice to improve bulbar function

Although there may be significant differences in practice between the United States and the United Kingdom, for example, this is not yet known.

The overall picture is that there is no general agreement as to the indications and safety of many of the procedures currently used in MND management, so that it is difficult to establish the principles of good practice in MND management (Table 12-4) Furthermore, it is almost impossible to adequately audit the quality of an MND service in a particular locality.

CONCLUSIONS

This brief review indicates that there are major methodological problems in the evaluation of bulbar symptoms in MND. Properly evaluated assessment tools do not, in general, exist. As a result, there are major difficulties with assessing the value of both possible "curative" treatment regimens and the various techniques used in everyday practical management.

REFERENCES

1. Newrick PG, Langton Hewer R. Motor neurone disease: can we do better? A study of 42 patients.*Br Med J* 1984;289:539–42.
2. Wade DT, Langton Hewer R, Skilbeck CE, David RM. *Stroke. A critical approach to diagnosis, treatment and management.* London: Chapman Hall, 1985.
3. Langton Hewer R. Is neurological disability and handicap measurable? In: *The management of the neurological patient.* Warlow C, Garfield J, eds. London: Churchill Livingstone, 1987:
4. Enderby PM. *The Frenchay dysarthria assessment.*San Diego: College Hill Press, 1983.

5. Tikofsky RS. Phonetic characteristics of dysarthria. PHS Research Grant N.B. 02221: 14, 1965.
6. Yorkston K, Beukelman D. A clinician-judged technique for quantifying dysarthric speech based on single word intelligibility. *J Comm Dis* 1980;13:15–31.
7. Plaitakis A, Smith J, Mandeli J, Yahr MD. Pilot trial of branched-chain aminoacids in amyotrophic lateral sclerosis. *Lancet* 1988;1:1015–8.
8. Norris FH, Smith RA, Denys EH. Motor neurone disease: towards better care. *Br Med J* 1985;291:259–62.
9. Enderby PM, Langton Hewer R. Communication and swallowing. In: Cochrane GM, ed. *The management of motor neurone disease.* London: Churchill Livingstone, 1987:
10. Mills CP. Dysphagia in pharyngeal paralysis treated by cricopharyngeal sphincterotomy. *Lancet 1973;1:455–7.*
11. Lebo CP, U KS, Norris FH. Cricopharyngeal myotomy in amyotrophic lateral sclerosis. *Laryngoscope* 1976; 86:862–8.
12. Loizou LA, Small M, Dalton GA. Cricopharyngeal myotomy in MND. *J Neurol Neurosug Psychiatry* 1980;34:42–5.
13. Mady S. Surgey for dysphagia in motor neuron disease. In: Rose FC, ed. *Research progress in motor neurone disease. London: Pitman, 1984:*
14. David VC. Relief of dysphagia in MND. with cricopharyngeal myotomy. *Ann R Coll Sur Eng* 1985;229–31.
15. Perry AR, Gawel M, Rose FC. Communication aids in patients with motor neurone disease. *Br Med J* 1981;282:1690–2.
16. Enderby P, ed. *Assistive Communication Aids.* London: Churchill Livingstone; 1987.
17. Saunders C, Walsh TD, Smith M. Hospice care in motor neurone disease. In: *Hospice — the living idea.* Arnold: Sanders, Summers and Teller, 1981:

Amyotrophic Lateral Sclerosis,
edited by F. Clifford Rose.
Demos Publications, New York © 1990.

13

Assessment of Dysphagia in Motor Neuron Disease

Catherine Jones

Charing Cross Hospital, London, England

Although bulbar symptoms may present as the initial signs in only 20–30% of motor neuron disease (MND) patients, the great majority will have developed them by the terminal stages. Progressive difficulty in communicating, often resulting in anarthria, can be both frustrating and socially isolating for the patient. This is frequently compounded by accompanying dysphagia, which can be life threatening as well as distressing for the patient and family.

The three aims of the study reported in this chapter are: (a) to evaluate the nature of dysphagia in MND, (b) to evaluate whether a clinical speech therapy examination of dysphagia can predict the outcome of the radiological barium swallow assessment, and (c) to evaluate the reliability of the patients' subjective account of their dysphagia.

SUBJECTS AND METHODS

In a pilot study, 20 patients with MND (13 men, 7 women) ages between 32 and 77 years (mean 55.6 years) were seen. Three assessments were carried out on each patient on the same day and were rated independently, viz.: (a) clinical speech therapy dysphagia assessment, (b) modified barium swallow assessment, and (c) subjective patient questionnaire.

In all three assessments, the swallowing sequence was divided into six functionally relevant headings and, under each heading, subtests were rated on a Yes/No scale; oral phase: (a) lips, (b) tongue and bolus control, (c) soft palate, and (d) trigger of swallow reflex; pharyngeal phase: (e) pharynx, and (f) aspiration.

In addition, the radiological assessment examined the esophageal phase and the speech therapy evaluation examined the functioning of the larynx.

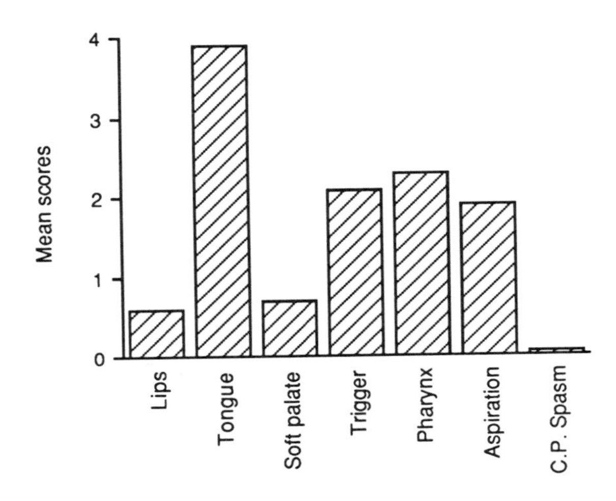

FIG 13-1. Pattern of impairment for 20 motor neuron disease patients.

RESULTS

Nature of Dysphagia

Radiological examination of the swallowing sequence in normals is divided into three phases—oral, pharyngeal, and esophageal. In this study, 11 motor neuron disease (MND) patients showed an abnormal oral phase, 7 showed a combined oral and pharyngeal abnormality, and 1 presented with isolated asymptomatic cricopharyngeal spasm as an esophageal disorder. No patient showed a pharyngeal abnormality in isolation.

Figure 13-1 shows the overall pattern of impairment for the 20 MND patients studied. The mean scores for each parameter of the swallow sequence is demonstrated. Tongue and bolus control was the most consistently severely impaired feature, often presenting as the only abnormality in mildly dysphagic patients. In severe cases, tongue movements were slow and laborious, with difficulty in moving the bolus posteriorly being magnified by a semisolid consistency. Liquid material was frequently lost into the anterior and lateral sulci, and consequently small amounts were not sufficient to trigger a swallow. Triggering of the swallow reflex, pharyngeal motility, and aspiration were the next cluster of features to be most consistently impaired. Aspiration was present in eight patients and in three of these aspiration was silent. Although appearance of the soft palate was abnormal in 18 patients and 5 showed asymptomatic nasal regurgitation, very few patients had regurgitation frequent or functionally sufficient enough to be scored as severe. Cricopharyngeal spasm occurred in one patient. Figure 13-2 shows the pattern of impairment in eight patients who presented initially with bulbar signs, and Fig. 13-3 shows the pattern in six

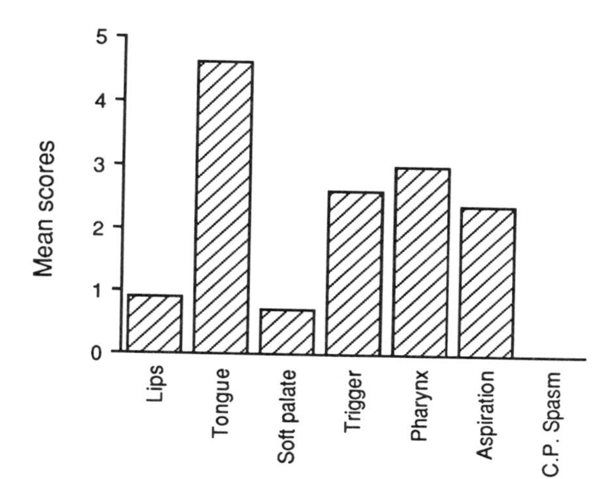

FIG 13-2. Pattern of impairment in eight MND patients who presented initially with bulbar signs.

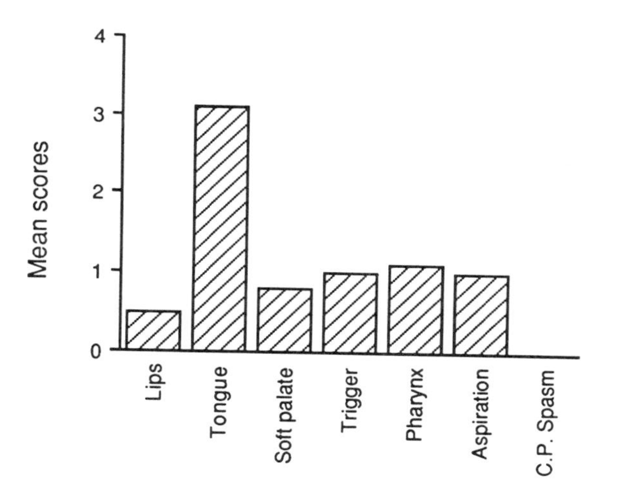

FIG 13-3. Pattern of impairment in six MND patients who presented with upper-limb signs.

Table 13-1. *Correlations of Totals*

	Radiology oral total	Radiology oral and pharyngeal total
Speech therapy oral total	0.6471 Sig. 0.002	0.7587 Sig. 0.000
Speech therapy oral & pharyngeal total	0.6295 Sig. 0.003	0.7203 Sig. 0.000

patients who presented with upper limb signs. The profiles are similar, with tongue and bolus control being the most severely abnormal feature, but the upper limb group show a less severe pattern overall than the bulbar group did.

Table 13-2. *Correlations of Speech Therapy and Radiology Subtests*

	Radiology subtests					
Speech therapy subtests	B1	B2	B3	B4	B5	B6
A1	0.6154 Sig. 0.004					
A2		0.5726 Sig. 0.008				
A3			0.3288 Sig. 0.157			
A4				0.1727 Sig. 0.467		
A5					0.234 Sig. 0.321	
A6						4921 Sig. 0.028

Table 13-3. *Correlation of Speech Therapy Total and Radiology Subtests*

	Radiology subtests					
	B1	B2	B3	B4	B5	B6
Speech therapy totals	.4793 Sig 0.032	.6145 Sig 0.004	.4966 Sig 0.026	.5394 Sig 0.014	.4284 Sig 0.059	.6885 Sig 0.001

Predictions from a Speech Therapy Assessment for the Radiological Results

Table 13-1 shows the correlations and significance levels of the speech therapy assessment with the radiological assessment split into oral, and oral and pharyngeal totals. The significance level suggests a strong positive correlation such that a patient scoring highly on one test will score highly on the other and vice versa.

Table 13-2 shows the correlation between individual subtests of the lips, tongue, and aspiration, suggesting that the speech therapy assessment has significant predictive value on these subtests. However, speech therapy assessment of the soft palate, the triggering of the swallow reflex, and the pharynx is a poor predictor of the corresponding radiological results.

Table 13-3 shows the combined total of the speech therapy subtests correlated with individual radiological subtests. A predictive value from the speech therapy assessment is seen with all radiological subtests apart from the pharynx.

Table 13-4 takes subtests from both the speech therapy and subjective patient assessment that were of highest predictive value and correlates the total with the radiological subtest of aspiration. This combination of clinical subtests would seem to be a good predictor of aspiration as measured radiologically.

At present, interjudge and intertest reliability measures are still being taken and, until completed, these results should be interpreted only tentatively.

Table 13-4. *Correlation of Selected Speech Therapy and Subjective Assessment Subtests with Radiological Aspiration*

		Radiology aspiration
Total speech therapy	Lips Tongue Trigger Aspiration	0.7282 Sig 0.000
Subject assessment	Tongue	

Table 13-5. *Correlation of Patient Subjective Assessment and Radiology Subtests*

	Subjective Subtests					
Radiology Subtests	C1	C2	C3	C4	C5	C6
B1	0.3903 Sig 0.089					
B2		0.6100 Sig.0.004				
B3			0.4338 Sig 0.056			
B4				0.4605 Sig 0.041		
B5					0.4707 Sig 0.036	
B6						0.2459 Sig. 0.0296

Reliability of Patients Account of Their Dysphagia

Table 13-5 shows the correlations and significance levels between individual subtests on the subjective patient assessment and the same subtests on radiological assessment. Patient assessment of tongue and bolus control and also of the pharynx shows a good predictive value for the radiological results. Awareness of pharyngeal abnormalities was shown by patients' complaints of food sticking in the throat or needing to wash down solid food with liquid. Patients appear unable to predict other features of the swallow sequence, and awareness of aspiration is noticeably poor.

CONCLUSIONS

Abnormal tongue and bolus control is the most consistently severely impaired feature of the swallow sequence. Pharyngeal disorders do not occur in isolation but may accompany the oral phase abnormality. Cricopharyngeal spasm appears infrequently in MND.

A clinical speech therapy assessment may predict the radiological outcome on certain features of the swallow sequence. The ability to predict aspiration is of particular importance, and it is hoped that results of this pilot study will lead to further development of the test to provide a reliable guide to clinicians. Because rapid deterioration can occur in MND, a clinical tool allowing reliable, economical, and regular reassessment may have considerable implications for management. Patients' accounts of their dysphagia should always be accompanied by detailed observations of them eating and drinking.

Acknowledgments: We are grateful to the Motor Neuron Disease Association for financing this project and also to the departments of radiology, neurology, ENT, and speech therapy for their cooperation and support.

REFERENCES

1. Gubbay S, Kahana E, Zilber N, et al. Amyotrophic lateral sclerosis. A study of its presentation and prognosis. *J Neurol* 1985; 232:295–300.
2. Price G, Jones C, Charlton R, et al. A combined approach to the assessment of neurological dysphagia. *Clin Otolaryngol* 1987; 12:197–201.

Amyotrophic Lateral Sclerosis,
edited by F. Clifford Rose.
Demos Publications, New York © 1990.

14

Electromyographic Assessment in Amyotrophic Lateral Sclerosis

Paolo Pinelli and [1]Fabrizio Pisano

First Neurological Clinic, University of Milan, St. Paolo Teaching Hospital, Milano, and [1]Department of Neurology, Medical Center of Rehabilitation, Clinica del Lavoro Foundation, Institute of Care and Research, Veruno, Italy

Several electromyographic (EMG) studies have been carried out in amyotrophic lateral sclerosis (ALS) that evaluated the natural course of the disease and the effects of treatments (1,2). Thus, several points of physiopathological interest have been assessed in a more quantitative way than possible with clinical investigation. Moreover, further changes induced by the pathological process can be foreseen with more suitable and appropriate EMG methods.

It is the main goal of the present chapter to analyze the ways by which we could detect the subclinical early motor unit (MU) alterations and to describe the most reliable procedures for a quantitative measurement of the course of motor disorders.

The electrophysiological criteria that can help identify the different levels on which treatments can impinge include psychological engagement as well as alterations of the upper (UMN) and lower (LMN) motor neurons.

INSTRUMENTATION

Recording Electrodes for EMG

The study of single MU activity has been carried out using different types of electrodes from the usual monopolar concentric needle electrodes (Disa 13 L 49/51). Surface (Disa 13 L 26/27, Disa 13 K 60) or Basmajan (Disa 13 K 71) electrodes have been used for very severely paretic muscles, but single fiber needle electrodes (Disa 13 K 87) are needed for a more detailed investigation of apparently normal muscles. In the latter case simultaneous double recordings have been carried out with "global" electrodes from the same muscle to better define the order of recruitment of the MU under study.

Amplifiers of two-channel EMG Medelec Mystro Plus have been employed.

METHODS

The measurement of interspike intervals (ISI) was made manually in the early phase of research, whereas a computerized system was adopted later. For each single experiment the impulse elicited in 60 s were acquired and sampled at a 1KHz rate, the EMG signal being converted to a digital shape. The elaboration program identified a trigger signal for each MU action potential (ap) and then measured the ISI. From these values the mean frequency, the ISI histogram, and the scatter diagram were calculated. The maximal voluntary contraction test (MVC) was carried out for 60 s, three times, under audiovisual feedback as described in a previous report (3).

The force was measured through transducers applied to a standardized point of the limb during isometric contraction. The measurements of fasciculation aps were performed with surface electrodes placed on corresponding agonistic and antagonistic muscles at the opposite sides of the arms and legs (4,5), the recordings being carried out for a period of 5 min at low speed.

The pharmacological assessment of MU function was performed by repeating the MVC tests after placebo and after 2 mg TRH-T i.m., for a period of at least 45 min.

SUBJECTS

The investigations were performed in 68 MUs of 4 muscles (biceps brachii, first dorsal interosseous, rectus femori, abductor hallucis brevis) of 6 normal subjects and in 164 MUs of the same muscles of 42 patients affected by ALS.

RESULTS

The MU changes detected in ALS can be subdivided into seven types described in the following paragraphs.

Signs of MU Early Disorder (First Stage)

The distribution of paresis in early and intermediate phases of ALS is very asymmetric and uneven in different muscles, which allows us to investigate the possible early signs of MU alteration in clinically normal muscles of patients diagnosed with ALS; we can then follow up the course of pathological process until complete paralysis. In the first phase, the lesion affects only a part of the motor neurons innervating a single muscle; the affected MUs (sick MUs) remain vital and capable of a certain degree of activity. The sick MU will die only after a certain span of time, which seems to last several months (1). So that the earliest abnormal effect of the disease will correspond to a functional change of a sick but still active MU. We name this stage of the disease, in which the only abnormality is represented by the presence of some sick MUs, the first stage. The following signs of MU sickness can be identified.

With reference to the neuroanatomical aspects of MU sickness, we have to consider the internal variability occurring in a volley of the MU aps. The values of duration, amplitude, and shape of the ap of the single MU are still within the normal range, but their variability in the volley of discharges is significantly increased. The assessment of this change can be carried out through two different methods that preferably should be associated: (a) global recording (with Basmajan electrode) to avoid as much as possible the influence of small occasional displacements of the electrode on the active electrical field entering the range of detection of the ap, (b) the single-fiber investigation for the occurrence of changes in jitter and block of transmission: the results of this investigation can further support the real "internal variability" of the MU ap. These changes can be considered a sign of a dying-back process depending on a more proximal alteration at the level of the neurotubular system and neurofilaments or of the neuronal soma.

It is likely that in this early phase some changes in the resting potential of the terminal branches of the LMN give rise to ectopic excitation responsible for fasciculation potentials that present with normal parameters. They can be clinically observed as small twitches that appear as a less frequent event than the spontaneous MU ap detected by EMG. The internal variability of such potentials is somewhat small. Repetitive discharges of voluntarily activated MUs, as doublets or multiplets, are a frequent finding as well as for spontaneous MU ap.

The histopathological changes of the neuronal soma are well documented: signs of atrophy with decrease in receptors, "ballooniform" changes, and dendritic alterations. These modifications can produce an ephatic cross excitation and a decrease in excitability with repercussion on MU recruitment and firing. The functional consequences are complicated by the associated alteration of the UMN, which can also impair the recruitment and firing of the corresponding MUs. The preliminary step for studying these impairments is represented by the identification of the range of normal variability of recruitment in standard condition of MVC. As a result of EMG study of the different types of MUs, we have required the following "minimal criteria of abnormality." The lowest limit of normality for the firing frequency corresponds to that of type S MU and for fatigability to that of type FF MUs. The parameters considered are: MU activation time, maximal firing frequency at the onset ($F_{o}mx$), maximal firing frequency at a certain time x ($F_{x}mx$), the histograms of ISI, the endurance (E) for MVC, and the range of MVS recruitment threshold (RR) at

RIGHT EXTENSOR DIGITORUM BREVIS

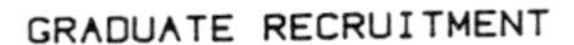

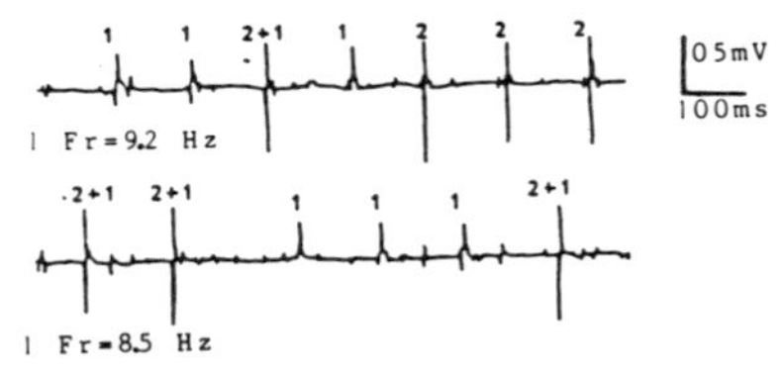

1) MINIMAL RECRUITMENT

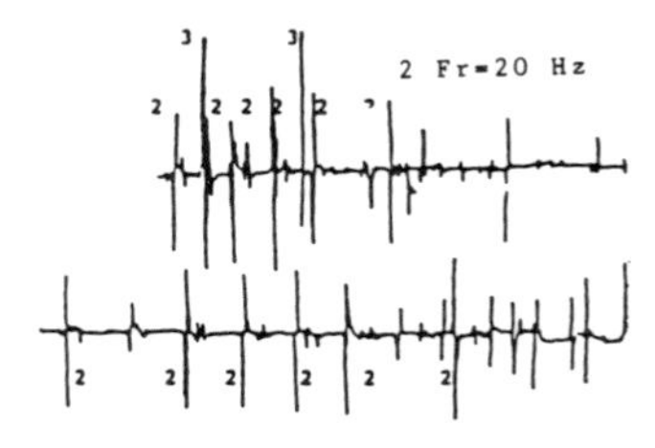

2) MODERATE RECRUITMENT

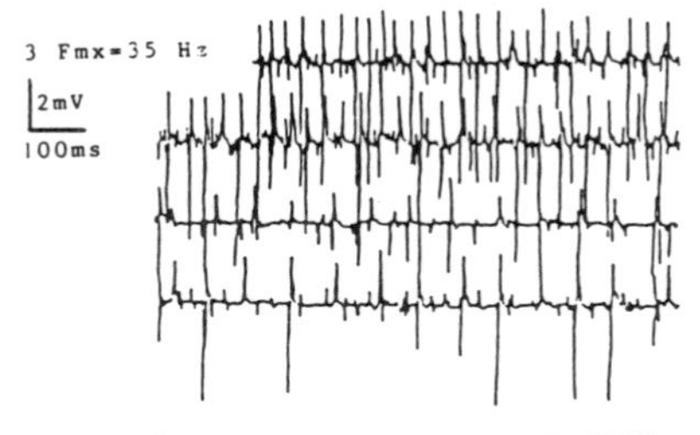

3) MAXIMAL RECRUITMENT

FIG.14-1. Recruitment and firing in lower motor neuron lesions. The occurrence of synchronous action potentials of motor unit (mu) 1 and 2 (2 + 1) was evaluated on higher speed tracing. 1): Minimal graduated effort and recruitment frequency (Fr) of the first MU when the second MU appears, 2): moderate graduated effort and Fr of the second MU, 3): maximal voluntary contraction. The calibration is changed from 0.5 to 2 mV.

graduated voluntary contraction. Further data can be collected in synchronized EMG with the analysis of two MU spike intervals (2SI). The main changes that can be found more often in UMN and LMN alterations are given in Figs. 14-1 and 14-2 and in Table 14-1. For ISI we refer particularly to the regularity of the ISIs, which are maintained relatively constant.

Random Denervated Muscle Fibers (Second Stage)

When a previously normal MU dies, the muscle fibers of its muscular unit (MuU) show, after a few weeks, fibrillation potentials occurring at the needle electrode insertion, and spontaneously picking-up such aps at this stage appears to be a tantalizing task because the denervated muscle fibers are

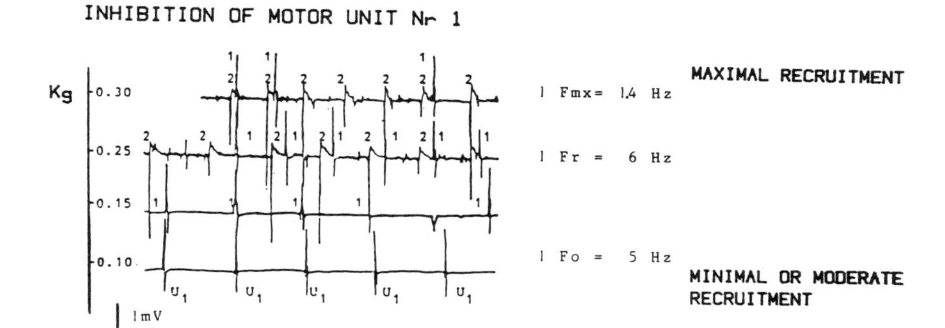

FIG. 14-2. Recruitment and firing in upper motor neuron lesions. On the ordinate axis, the output force was measured on the dorsal aspect of the second finger. At maximal output force, the firing frequency on the second motor unit (MU) increases whereas the firing of the first MU is inhibited. F_o, frequency of firing at minimal voluntary effort; Fr, frequency of firing at the first MU when the second MU fires at F_o; Fmx, frequency of firing at maximal voluntary effort.

randomly distributed among normal ones in a large area of muscle. Global electrodes such as the Basmajan electrodes are more suitable, but a high gain of the amplifier is required because of their low impedance. Previous stimulation of the muscle with long-lasting (50ms) electrical impulses may enhance the occurrence of the fibrillation potentials. An alternative expedient is the injection of an anticholinesterase drug, e.g., neostigmine, which exerts a more delayed effect.

Enlargement of the Surviving MUs (Third Stage)

The surviving normal MUs are able to reinnervate the "orphan" denervated muscle fibers, i.e., the so called "collateral sprouting" phenomenon (CS). The

TABLE 14-1. *Schematic Representation of Changes in the Variables of Single Motor Unit (MU) Firing in the Maximal Voluntary Contraction Test: Maximal Firing at Onset ($F_o$mx), Regularity of Interspike Intervals (ISI), Maximal Firing at Time x ($F_x$mx), Endurance (E), Threshold of Recruitment of Successive MUs (RR), and Reciprocal Intervals of Spikes of Two MUs (2SI), in Lower Motor Neuron (LMN) and Upper MN (UMN) Lesions*

	$F_o$mx	ISI	RR	$F_x$mx	E	2SI
LMN	—	↑	↑	—	Å	—
UMN	↓	↓	↓	↓	—	↓

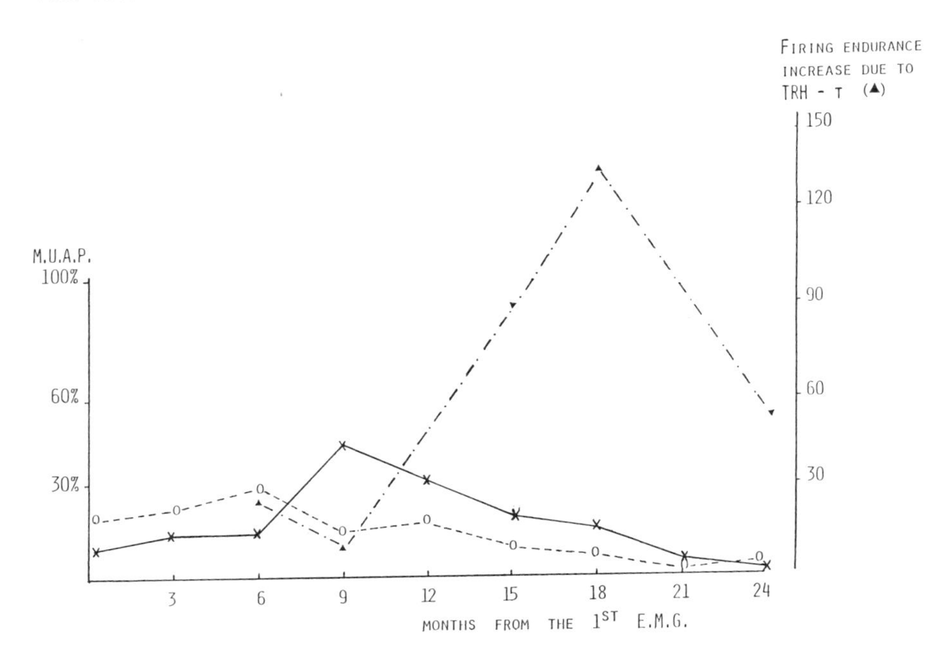

FIG.14-3. M.A.-A.L.S.-biceps brachii muscle. On the left ordinate: the percentage of MUaps with increased duration and linked potentials (x) and of M.U.A.P. with increased amplitude ○ evaluated every 3 months during a period of 24 months (on the abscissa). On the right ordinate: the percentage increased in endurance of firing of single MUs after the acute TRH-T test (▲) on the 6th, 9th, 15th, 18th, and 24th month.

identification of this process can be carried out with a statistical study of the percentage of giant MU aps (GMU) with respect to the total number of sampled MU aps. In a previous report (6), on the basis of changes in MU aps, according to the principle adopted by Buchthal, we identified three different groups of MU in the biceps brachii muscle of four ALS patients. The first group included normal values of duration and amplitude. The second group was characterized by increased duration (+25%) of the main phase and/or increased number and amplitude (25% of the main phase) of linked potentials (L). The third group of MU aps had an increased amplitude (> 3 mV). The percentage of MU ap, group 2 and 3 with respect to the total number of MU aps (at least 10), was taken into account as an index of sprouting. Only muscles with a preserved total number of recruitable MUs of at least 10 were included in this follow-up study.

In Fig. 14-3 we can see the percentage changes in MU aps with increased duration and L, and in MU aps with increased amplitude. In the same diagram the percentage changes in MU responsivity for endurance to TRH-T acute test is also shown. There is evidence of a significant increase in MU aps percentage with increased duration and L that occurred between the 6th and the 9th months from the first EMG evaluation. It also appears that the collateral sprouting is mainly of the "dispersed" type because it affects the duration more than the amplitude. On the other hand, the impairment of endurance, partially responsive to TRH, occurs later towards the 15th–18th month.

The analysis of the "internal variability" of the single MU aps can yield useful data regarding the dating of the CS. Early (or nascent) GMUs are characterized by a normal initial spike, with later components as linked potentials whose occurrence in the volley is somewhat inconstant. This variability inside the MU ap disappears in the stage of mature–normal GMU. A further finding indicative of the site of CS in the nerve fiber of ALS patients with respect to the site of CS in acquired neuropathies is represented by the absence of axon reflexes in ALS. This means that CS occurs only at the intramuscular level in ALS patients, whereas it originates more proximally at an extramuscular level in acquired neuropathies.

Late Dying GMUs (Fourth Stage)

The neuropathy of ALS at this stage can also affect the GMUs. The signs of sickness of the GMUs is represented by an increase in the internal variability of the GMU ap also affecting the first spike. Moreover, these GMUs can undergo ectopic hyperexcitability; as a consequence, fasciculations with large twitches and GMU aps represent a typical finding at this stage.

Loss of Recruitable MUs

No block of conduction has been ascertained in ALS and, apart from the functional impairments previously described, the loss of force is due to a Wallerian-like degeneration of the MUs. In some phases a MU is discharging ectopically, although it is not recruited by voluntary effort.

The best quantitative evaluation of the remaining vital MUs seems to be represented by the measurements of force associated with the recording of the convolute EMG at MVC. The measurement of the area of the Mmx response for comparison can also offer an index of the loss of MU recruitment due to UMN impairment.

The more recent electromagnetic transcranial stimulation does not add reliable information to the amount of the population of MNs.

A Supplementary Evaluation of the First, Third, and Fourth Stages: the TRH Test

TRH is known to increase the rate of firing frequency and the duration of response of the LMNs to descending glutamergic corticospinal impulses. The gain setting effect of TRH is state dependent and it has been shown to occur in some sick MNs (7), concerning particularly parameters such as E, and F MX

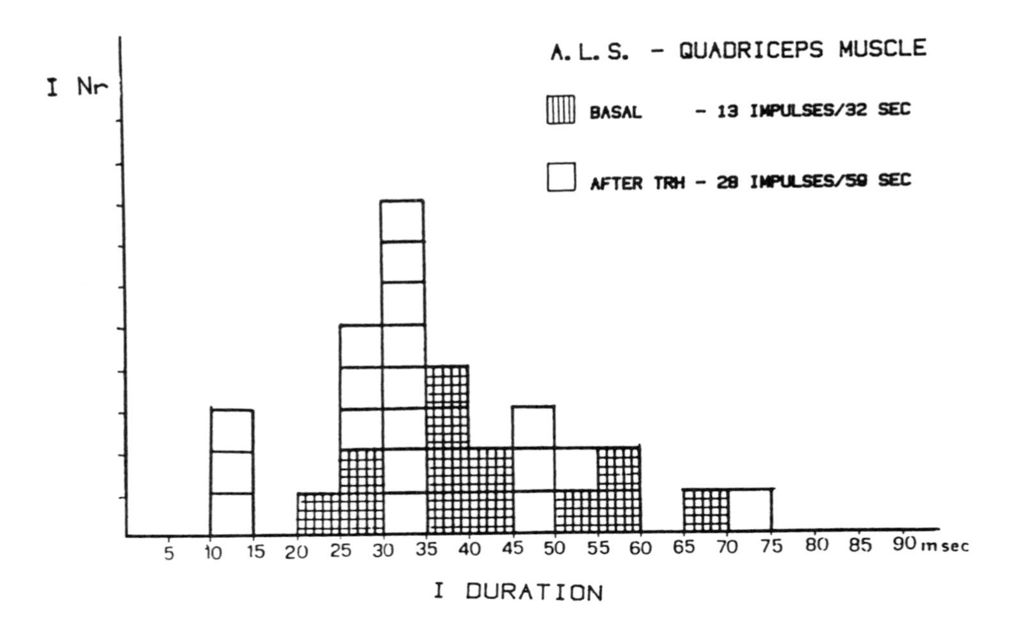

FIG.14-4. Interspike intervals of one motor unit discharging during maximal voluntary contraction in basal conditions and after TRH.

(Fig. 4). The occurrence of double discharges in the middle of the 60 min MVC test can also be increased.

Some Objective Criteria About the Level of Changes in Recruitment

It is obvious that the changes described in the paragraphs above can be due only to intrinsic changes at the peripheral level, "inside" the MUs, without any subjective factor from the patient's attitude. On the contrary, the changes that can occur in MU recruitment in MVC, as far as they include the voluntary effort, may depend on different mechanisms operating from the psychological as well as the spinal level.

We will indicate the increase in recruited MUs as Nx → Nx + 1 MUs factor. Consistent differences can be shown by the functional EMG according to the psychological or spinal mechanisms causing Nx → Nx + 1. The parameters considered regard the F mx and Fr (recruitment frequency, that is the firing frequency of Nx when Nx + 1 is first recruited) in different, well-identified conditions of voluntary contraction. Changes in voluntary effort affect the value of Fr in the sense that if the subject increases the voluntary effort, Fr will increase towards the F mx value and Nx → Nx + 1 will occur. If there is an increase Nx → Nx + 1 while the Fr of the MU Nx is still low, there is evidence that something has improved at a neurophysiological level, possibly operating at the spinal level (increase in LMN response). On the other hand, a change in voluntary effort cannot modify Fr. In conclusion, if Nx → Nx + 1 occurs with a Fr that is <F mx, this represents good evidence for a "spinal" effect.

CONCLUSIONS

For the practical evaluation of previously described methods, several criteria are needed: a) how easily they can be applied; b) their reliability and meaning for the identification of functional changes; c) the relationship with the main clinical aspects of the ongoing disorder. As shown in the EMG, the finding of GMUs ap typical for CS represents a consistent advantage offered by the most traditional and universally accepted EMG methodology. On the other hand, we have found that it is possible to develop a statistical quantitative evaluation of the CS during long periods of the disease. It can also be related to measurements of force to evaluate how much the CS can induce some improvement during the natural course of the disease. Obviously, the real GMU must be differentiated from the polyphasic MU ap that is due to slowing of conduction in the terminal branches of a sick MU. The investigations reported above can help recognize the role played by such "sickness." Moreover, the TRH acute test can be added as a useful complementary investigation of a possible degree of reversibility of the functional impairment and particularly of the abnormal fatigability of the sick MUs with reference not only to the LMN but also to the UMN.

The evaluation of Nx → Nx + 1 with the criteria reported in the section on objective criteria for levels of changes in recruitment may be of great significance when considered in the frame of measurements of the total population of MUs (5). In fact, the recruitment of new MUs is the most consistent change able to affect the motor performances of the patient.

REFERENCES

1. Mazzarello P, Pasetti C, Pinelli P, Poloni M, Villani A. Towards a definition of neuronopathic process in ALS: the staging of electromyographic findings. In: Pinelli P, Pasetti A, Mora G, eds. *Neurophysiological contributions for assessing rehabilitation in lower and upper motorneuron diseases.* Padova: Liviana Press, 1984:97:115.
2. Swash M, and Schwartz MS. Staging MND: single fibre EMG studies of asymmetry, progression and compensatory reinnervation. In: Rose FC, ed. *Research progress in MND.* London: Pitman, 1984;123–40.
3. Pinelli P, Pisano F, Crespi B. Il reclutamento delle unita motorie nelle amiotrofie neurogene. In: Franchignoni FP, ed. *Interventi riabilitativi nelle malattie neuromuscolari.* Veruno:Alganon, 1986:3–20.
4. Norris FH Jr. Adult spinal motor neuron disease. Progressive muscular atrophy

(Aran's disease) in relation to amyotrophic lateral sclerosis. In: Vinken PJ, Bruyn GW, eds. *System disorders atrophies,* 1975: (Handbook of clinical neurology; vol 22.)
5. Roth G. Fasciculations d'origine périphérique. *Electromyography* 1971;11:413–28.
6. Pinelli P, Pasetti C, Mazzini L, Pisano F, Villani A. Motorneuron sprouting and spinal plasticity in amyotrophic lateral sclerosis: the "window of opportunity" for a ganglioside treatment. In: Tettamanti G, Ledeen RW, Sandhoff K, Nagai Y, Toffano G, eds. *Gangliosides and neuronal plasticity* Padova: Liviana Press, 1986:543–60.
7. Pinelli P. *Dall'ultima unità motoria alla volontà.* Catania: Ed. TB Today, Cyanamid, 1988.

Amyotrophic Lateral Sclerosis,
edited by F. Clifford Rose.
Demos Publications, New York © 1990.

Electromyographic Monitoring and Prognostication in Amyotrophic Lateral Sclerosis

Eric H. Denys

ALS and Neuromuscular Research Center,
Pacific Presbyterian Medical Center,
San Francisco, California, U.S.A.

In amyotrophic lateral sclerosis (ALS) two counteractive forces are at work: denervation and reinnervation. These can be assessed by means of a needle electrode examination during electromyographic (EMG) testing. Progression of the disease will depend on the net excess force and can be documented easily; lack of progression could similarly be substantiated and be very valuable in judging the effect of new treatment modalities. The role of EMG in predicting the course of the disease is more difficult to assess. In this study, the EMG records of deceased patients were reviewed, and predictions of survival were made on the basis of a single study without knowledge of the subsequent course of the disease. With some exceptions, a slow (over 36 months disease duration), average (24–36 months), or fast course (less than 24 months) could be predicted.

EMG plays an essential role in establishing the diagnosis of ALS. Besides the clinical examination, the EMG is undoubtedly the single most valuable diagnostic test. Once the diagnosis is established, repeat examinations are infrequently performed because of the inherent discomfort for the patient, and perhaps more importantly, because of the lack of therapeutic decisions based on the EMG findings.

Although EMG information has been obtained in patients in different stages of the disease, longitudinal studies have rarely been carried out; this is unfortunate when one realizes that the EMG gathers information about the underlying disease processes of denervation and reinervation that cannot be obtained in any other way. Moreover, repeat EMGs can document unquestionable progression of the disease by showing increasing denervation or

Table 15-1. *Electromyographic Documentation of Progressing Amyotrophic Lateral Sclerosis (55-Year-Old Patient with History of 4 Mo Dysarthria, Arm Fatigue, Hyperactive Reflexes, Tongue Fibrillations)*

	EMG at 4 M	8 M[a]	11 M
Rt. masseter	0|+|0[b]		
Rt. tongue	0|+|0		
1st. D.I.O.	0|0|0	0|+|+++	++|++|+++
Rt. ext. dig. com.	0|0|+	0|0|+++	++|++|+++
Rt. deltoid	0|0|+	0|0|+++	0|+|+++
Rt. ant. tib.	0|0|0	0|0|++	0|+|++
Rt. gast. med.	0|0|0	0|0|++	+|++|++
Lt. ext. dig. com.	+|+|+++	0|++|++	
Norris Scale (5)	87	88	73

[a] On pyridostigmine.
[b] Positive sharp waves/fibrillations/fasciculations.

involvement of previously normal muscles, as shown in Table 15-1; the corollary, lack of progression, could similarly be demonstrated and would be a very valuable tool in experimental treatment trials.

Although ALS is characterized by a combination of denervation and reinervation, striking differences can be found between patients presenting clinically in a similar fashion. It could be postulated that the rate of disease progression will be determined primarily by the net effects of these two counteractive forces, with upper motor neuron involvement playing a secondary role. It is therefore tempting to try to predict the course of the disease on the basis of EMG findings obtained at one particular moment. To evaluate this hypothesis, EMG records of patients studied 10 years ago were reviewed for analysis.

MATERIALS AND METHODS

Only patients with an unequivocable clinical and electromyographic diagnosis of ALS and clinical follow-up data until the time of death were included in this analysis. This group consisted of 21 patients, 11 men ages 48–71 years (mean = 61) and 10 women, ages 42–82 years (mean = 59). Nerve conduction studies were normal in all or were consistent with changes seen in motor neuron disease.

In all patients, needle electrode examination had been performed by means of a concentric needle electrode and the findings were tabulated in a standardized fashion; positive sharp waves and fibrillations were each reported on a scale of 0 to ++++ and were quantitated as

0 = none detected
+ = detected in at least two areas, but searching is necessary
++ = readily present in several areas of the muscle
+++ = discharges persisting for some time after needle movement
++++ = virtually continuous fibrillation potentials and positive sharp waves

Motor unit potential (MUP) analysis included a description of the degree of motor unit loss and the number of increased-duration MUPs. Long-duration, polyphasic MUPs reflecting reinnervation were commonly found; there were instances, however, in which large reinnervation MUPs were much more abundantly present and this had been noted in the records. In some instances reinnervation was virtually absent and this had similarly been recorded. All studies were performed by the same examiner.

For the purpose of this analysis, an estimate of denervation activity per extremity was arrived at by giving a value of +, ++, or +++ based on positive sharp waves and fibrillations combined in extremities where at least three muscles were examined. An estimate of reinnervation was expressed as slight, average, or marked, based on the examiner's written observations.

The time between onset of the first symptoms and the electromyographic study was expressed in months and a preliminary prediction of disease duration was made. Survival between 24 and 36 months was considered average; a disease course was designated fast, and >36 months slow. The records were subsequently reviewed for disease duration from the time of the first symptoms until the time of the EMG, and with this additional information an adjusted prediction was made.

RESULTS

The denervation activity represented in Table 15-2 reveals no striking differences between patients in different categories that would help predict the outcome. Reinnervation, on the other hand, could be used as a predictor; patients with little or no reinnervation had the shortest survival, whereas patients with more than average reinnervation had the longest survival. Of the patients with a predicted fast disease course, only one patient survived much longer than predicted (patient 5); onset of the disease was in the lower extremities and upper motor neuron signs were not particularly prominent. Two of the 10 patients with a predicted average course died after 11 months

Table 15-2. *Prediction of ALS Course on the Basis of Electromyographic (EMG) Data*

Patient/ Sex/Age(yr)	Denervation[b]	Re-innervation	Predict	Mos Before EMG	New Predict	Total Disease (mo)
1. M 65	++|+++	0	Fast	12	Fast	27
2. M 48	++|+++	Little	Fast	12	Fast	12
3. F 49	0|++	Little	Fast	2	Fast	13
4. M 71	0|++	Little	Fast	5	Fast	9
5. M 55	+|+++	0	Fast	20	Fast	40[a]
6. F 82	+|+|+	0	Avg.–Fast	12	Avg.–Fast	17
7. M 65	+|+++	+	Avg.	6	Avg.	27
8. F 68	+|+++|+++	+	Avg.	10	Avg.	30
9. M 64	+|+	+	Avg.	9	Avg.	30
10. F 55	+|++	+	Avg.	7	Avg.	11[a]
11. M 64	0|0|++	+	Avg.	9	Avg.	26
12. F 64	0|0|++|+++	0	Avg.	10	Avg.(UMN)	27
13. F 56	+|++	+	Avg.	4	Avg.	11[a]
14. M 58	+|++	+	Avg.	4	Avg.	26
15. M 58	+|++|++|+++	+	Avg.	5	Avg.	30
16. F 61	+|+++|+++	+	Avg.	16	Avg.	35
17. F 59	+|++	+	Avg.	25	Slow	47
18. F 53	+|++|++	+	Avg.–Slow	5	Avg.–Slow	48
19. M 58	0|0|+|+	+	Avg.–Slow	6	Avg.–Slow	74
20. M 67	+++|+++|+++	+	Avg.	72	Slow	92
21. F 42	+|++|++	+	Avg.	20	Slow	73

[a] Incorrect prediction. For details see text. UMN, upper motor neuron.
[b] Expressed as an estimate per extremity. For details, see text.

because they declined respiratory support; therefore, respiratory function, which can be selectively involved early on, needs to be taken into account in disease prognosis (see Discussion). The duration of disease before the EMG test is certainly of some value in predicting survival; i.e., when no reinnervation is taking place but the patient has already survived 20 months, one is most likely dealing with a moderate disease process (patient 5). Such course, however, would be difficult to anticipate when studying the patient after only 5 months of disease.

In the group of patients with a slow disease course, the 92-month survival of patient 20 is perhaps surprising in light of the significant denervation, yet in keeping with the hypothesis that the degree of reinnervation is a better predictor of disease. In this study, respirator dependence was used as an endpoint of disease; however, none of the patients with a long survival were ventilator-dependent.

Table 15-3. *Disease Duration Based on First Area of Involvement*

	Fast	Average	Slow
Bulbar	3	4	2
Upper extremity	1	—	1
Lower extremity	2	3	1
Upper motor neuron	—	3	1
Total	6	10	5

Analysis of disease duration based on the body part first affected failed to show any correlation (Table 15-3).

DISCUSSION

Predicting an average course should not be difficult in ALS, in which 50% of the patients die within 3 years, and indeed, the majority of patients fell into that group. More important is the ability to detect those individuals who will deviate from the norm. It is well known that patients presenting with progressive muscular atrophy or primarily lateral sclerosis have a much longer survival, but there is currently no way to predict which patients with classic ALS, i.e., with both upper and lower neuron involvement, will have a faster or slower than average course. A prognosis based on EMG data is therefore of interest.

The incorrect predictions warrant further comment. The categories of survival are obviously arbitrary and do not totally eliminate relatively small deviations as seen with the first patient in Table 15-2. Patient 5 should have been predicted to have at least an average course in light of the 20 months already elapsed by the time of the EMG evaluations; however, the lack of reinnervation at that time was interpreted to indicate that the disease might be taking a turn for the worse, which in retrospect it did not. The denervation process itself was therefore most likely progressing slowly. Although reinnervation seemed to correlate best with survival, it is possible that the reinnervation capacity is, in turn, dependent on the severity of the denervating process.

It is clear that information other than denervation/reinnervation such as pulmonary function and degree of upper motor neuron involvement could enhance prognostication. Respiratory failure can occur at any time and even be a presenting manifestation of ALS (1). A pulmonary function test is undoubtedly superior over an EMG to assess that aspect of the disease (2,3); patient 13 (Table 15-2), fell in this category of respiratory failure and declined life support. In patient 12 (Table 15-2), the prediction of an average rather than a fast course was made, despite the absence of reinnervation potentials, because of the presence of marked upper motor neuron involvement, reflected in the slow firing rate of the motor units. The total disease duration was indeed average (27 months).

In addition, although a prediction was attempted solely on the basis of the EMG findings at that time, the value of additional knowledge of disease duration before the test cannot be disregarded.

In this exercise in prognostication, a number of assumptions were made; it was assumed that differences in denervation and reinnervation could be identified and estimated, that the relative degree of denervation and reinnervation as it was found at the time of the EMG would continue to operate during the remainder of the disease, and that impaired function of the lower motor neuron plays a more important role than that of the upper motor neuron; clearly none of these are absolute. If a constant process were operating it could be postulated that the rate of clinical decline would be steady, as has been claimed (4). However, based on computer simulations (see Chapter 21), a steady rate of clinical decline does not necessarily mean that the denervation/reinnervation ratio remains the same throughout the course of the disease; indeed, if the dropout of motor neurons (denervation) were constant, remaining reinnervated units would eventually fail and, because of their large territory, cause rapidly increasing weakness and an accelerating course; this pattern of acceleration has been well demonstrated in some patients by means of longitudinal pulmonary function studies (2).

At the present time EMG remains an imperfect tool for assessing denervation. Experienced electromyographers will agree that abundant positive sharp waves and fibrillations can be encountered with little or no loss of strength and that initial large-amplitude sharp waves and fibrillations may become small and undetectable in chronic neurogenic disease.

The development of newer techniques such as single-fiber EMG and macro EMG, allowing measurement of fiber density and single motor unit amplitude, will provide a better estimate of reinnervation and could improve the predictive value of EMG (6). The measurement of firing frequencies would similarly allow the assessment of upper motor neuron involvement, especially because patients with predominantly upper motor neuron involvement have a more benign course.

Although prediction using standard techniques has proved to be fairly accurate, further study is clearly needed, particularly on a longitudinal basis and by means of more refined techniques.

Acknowledgment: The assistance of Linda Elias, R.N., for data retrieval is greatly appreciated. Supported by the ALS and Neuromuscular Research Foundation, 2351 Clay Street, #416, San Francisco, California 94115.

REFERENCES

1. Parhad IM, Clark AW, Barron KD, et al. Diaphragmatic paralysis in motor neuron disease. *Neurology* 1978; 28:12–22.
2. Fallat RJ, Jewitt B, Bass M, et al. Spirometry in amyotrophic lateral sclerosis. *Arch Neurol* 1979; 36:74–80.
3. Norris FH, Fallat RJ: Staging respiratory failure in ALS. Tsubaki T, Yase Y, eds. *Amyotrophic lateral sclerosis. Recent advances in research and treatment.* New York: Elsevier, 1988:217–22
4. Munsat TL, Andres PL, Finison L, et al. The natural history of motorneuron loss in amyotrophic lateral sclerosis. *Neurology* 1988; 38:409-13.
5. Norris FH, Calanchini PR, Fallat RJ, et al. The administration of guandine in amyotrphic lateral sclerosis. *Neurology* 1974; 24:721–8.
6. Stalberg E, Sanders DB. The motor unit in ALS studies with different neurophysiological techniques. In: Rose FC, ed. *Research progress in motor neurone disease.* London: Pitman; 1984:105–22.

Amyotrophic Lateral Sclerosis,
edited by F. Clifford Rose.
Demos Publications, New York © 1990.

16

Neurophysiological Monitoring in Amyotrophic Lateral Sclerosis

David A. Ingram

The London Hospital, London, England

Amyotrophic lateral sclerosis (ALS) is characterized by progressive degeneration and eventual cell death of motor neurons in central and peripheral motor pathways. This gives rise to a typical picture in which lower motor neuron signs of weakness, wasting, and fasciculation of affected muscles occurs in association with upper motor neuron signs of increased tone and hyper-reflexia. Hitherto the assessment and grading of these features during monitoring of the disease has relied largely on clinical measures.

These measures form the basis of the clinical scales described in detail elsewhere in this volume and provide data that has direct relevance to the patients' functional disability (1,2). However, the individual measures, for example manual evaluation of strength and reflexes, are often imprecise and depend on good inter-rater reliability. The cumulative scores provided by scales can be readily compared from one examination to the next and frequently show a linear decline at all rates of progression (2), but these global values may mask the often focal onset and asymmetrical nature of the disease (3,4). This is an important distinction because the factors that determine the rate of progression and the relative resistance of certain motor neuron pools (3) are currently not known, and further research is required in this area.

In advanced disease the peripheral component tends to predominate. This can make clinical assessment of the degree of central motor involvement difficult. Indeed, the Babinski response, usually the most reliable clinical measure of corticospinal disease, may prove impossible to elicit in the later stages.

Neurophysiological techniques provide an alternative means for quantifying abnormalities of motor function, especially as recent developments have provided new methods suitable for use in a clinical setting. These permit accurate and independent investigations of both central and peripheral motor

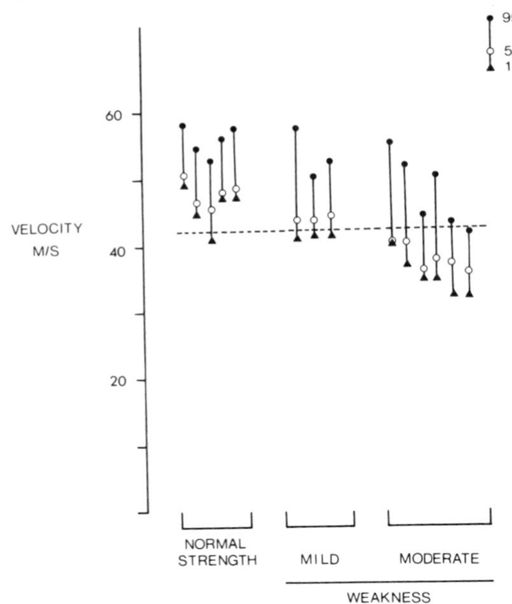

FIG. 16-1. Motor nerve conduction velocity ranges for the median nerve in 14 amyotrophic lateral sclerosis patients. Velocities for the fastest 5% (closed circles), slowest 5% (open circles), and slowest 1% (triangles) fibers are shown in each case. Patients with normal strength are compared with those presenting with mild (MRC grade 4) or moderate (MRC grade < 4) weakness of thenar abduction. The dotted line represents the lower limit of normal (mean -2 SD) for the slowest 1% fibers in normal control subjects.

conduction and are described below. Needle electromyographic techniques are considered by Pinelli elsewhere in this volume (Chapter 14).

PERIPHERAL MOTOR CONDUCTION

Conventional nerve conduction studies provide measurements of maximal velocities in motor nerves, and are usually normal in patients with ALS. In advanced disease with prominent muscle atrophy, mild slowing of maximal motor conduction velocity may occur in association with an increase in the distal motor latency (5). This reduction in velocity was initially attributed to preferential loss of the largest-diameter alpha motor neurons, the lower conduction velocity representing a normal sub-population of smaller-diameter and slower-conducting fibers (5,6), but it is now clear that pathological slowing of motor nerve conduction does occur in diseased neurons (7,8).

The degree of slowing can be monitored with a newly developed noninvasive technique (9) that accurately measures the entire range of motor conduction velocities (Fig. 16-1). Provided careful attention is paid to limb temperature, the maximum variability between investigations for any subpopulation of

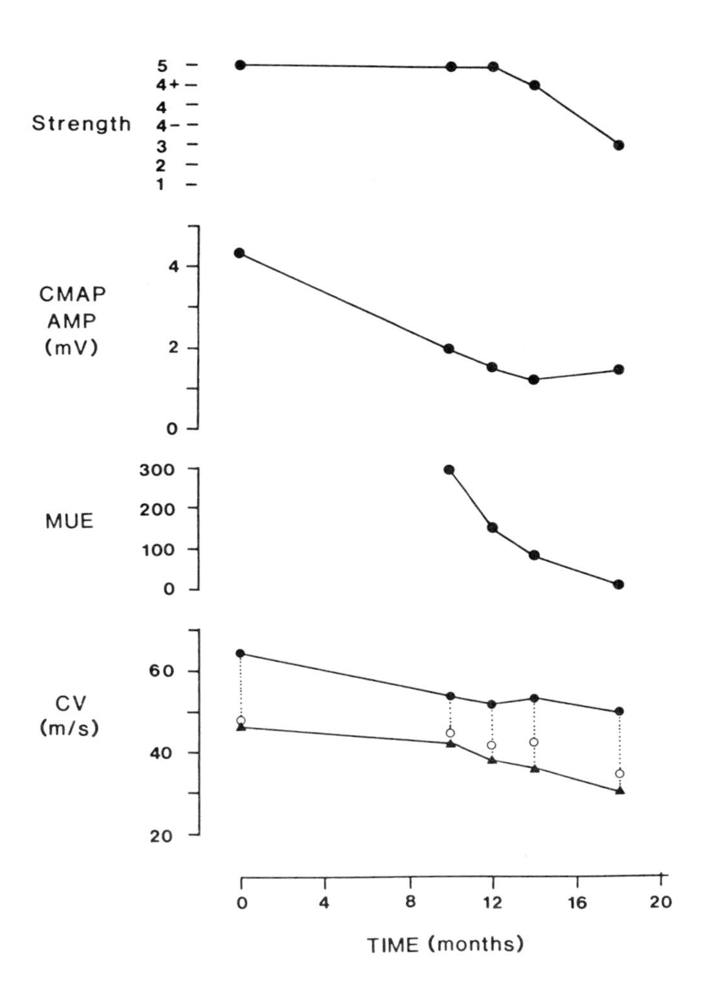

FIG. 16-2. Conduction velocity (CV) ranges for the median nerve in one amyotrophic lateral sclerosis patient during follow-up of 18 months (symbols as in Fig. 16-1). These are compared with strength (MRC grade), compound muscle action potential amplitude (CMAP AMP) and motor unit count (MUE) obtained from the thenar eminence.

neurons is <5.5% in normal nerves, which is in good agreement with the observations of Buchthal and Rosenfalck (10) on sensory neurons. The results in ALS indicate that the disease does not preferentially affect particular subpopulations of neurons and the reduction in velocity may exceed 30% of the initial value (Fig. 16-2).

These changes in conduction velocity can be shown in individual subjects to occur pari passu with the reduction in size of the functional motor neuron pool demonstrated by McComas and colleagues (11), and with a reduction in amplitude of the compound motor action potential (Fig. 16-2). There is a less exact relation to strength, measured by manual muscle testing, which probably reflects the compensatory effect of reinnervation in early stages of the disease (12). By applying the technique to different muscles in the same patient, it is also possible to examine the function of separate motor neuron pools, which allows further study of the asymmetry of the disease process.

Refractory period measurements have been reported to be abnormal in approximately one-third of alpha motor neurons in ALS (7), but this observation could not be confirmed using a noninvasive technique that accurately measures the range of refractory periods in motor nerves (8,13). The latter study showed that the refractory period of transmission for all alpha motor neurons remained within normal limits at all stages of the disease regardless of the rate of progression. However, there was agreement between the two studies in that refractory period measurements did not bear a consistent relationship to conduction velocity measurements, suggesting a mismatch in diseased neurons.

CENTRAL MOTOR CONDUCTION

Effective percutaneous stimulation of the brain in conscious subjects can now be achieved with two different techniques. In the first, introduced by Merton and Morton (14), electrical stimuli are directly applied to the scalp overlying the motor cortex. The brief, high-voltage capacitor discharges delivered by their device are capable of directly exciting descending motor pathways that control muscles in the contralateral arm and leg. The subject feels only minor discomfort and the muscle responses elicited by single stimuli are large, reproducible, and easily recorded using surface electrodes.

If the same stimuli are applied over the spinal column, peripheral nerve roots are excited near their exit foramina (15), which allows direct evaluation of the peripheral conduction time. By subtracting the peripheral conduction time from the motor latency after cortical stimulation, a measure of the central motor conduction time (CMCT) can be obtained. CMCT measurements represent the sum of the conduction time in the descending motor tracts, the activation time for alpha motor neurons, and the conduction time along the nerve roots. If stimuli of increased intensity are applied over the spine, descending motor tracts within the cord can be directly excited, which permits separate evaluation of cord conduction times. These can be expressed as a spinal conduction velocity (16).

The alternative technique (17) achieves effective brain and spinal column stimulation by means of brief time-varying magnetic pulses that induce small depolarizing currents within neural tissue. These stimuli are much better tolerated than electrical stimuli because they are virtually painless, and are also more effective due to the lack of attenuation of magnetic fields through body

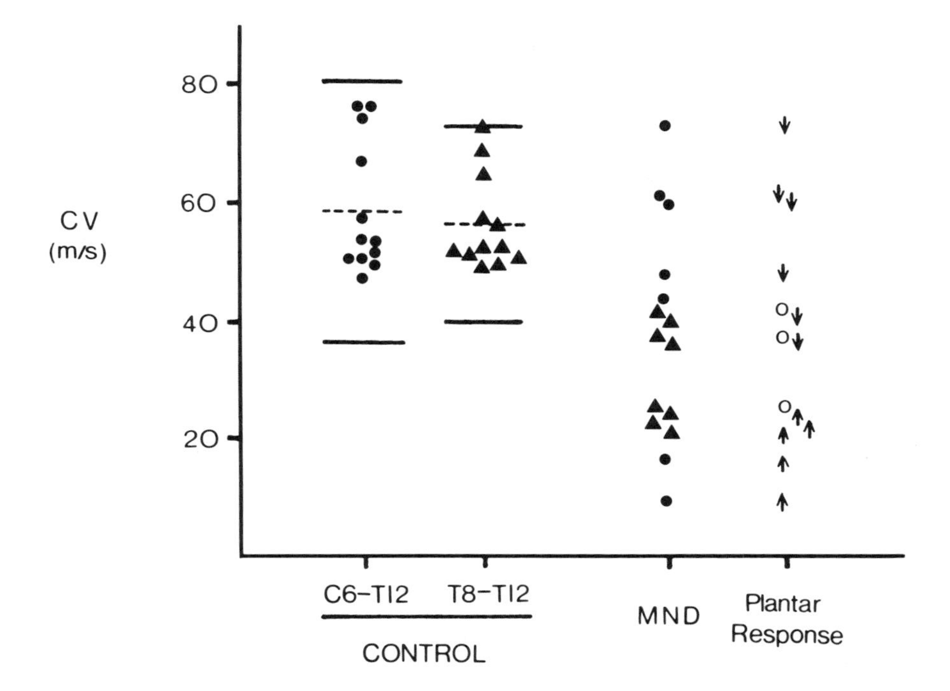

FIG. 16-3. Spinal motor conduction velocities for normal control subjects (closed circles C6–T12 segment; closed triangles T8–T12 segment) compared with equivalent values in amyotrophic lateral sclerosis (ALS) (MND) patients. In each ALS case the corresponding plantar response (↓,flexor;↑,extensor; o,unobtainable) is plotted to the right. There is a close relationship between the clinical and electrophysiological findings. Bars: mean ±2 SD. (Reproduced with permission from ref. 16.)

tissues and clothing. CMCT measurements can be obtained for arm and leg muscles in the same way as for electrical stimulation, but spinal conduction cannot be separately evaluated because magnetic stimuli are incapable of exciting motor tracts within the cord.

Abnormalities of central motor conduction have been demonstrated in ALS with both techniques (16, 18, 19). In studies with electrical stimulation (16, 19) it was generally more difficult to excite central motor pathways than in normal controls, a relative refractoriness not related to age but more prominent in advanced disease. Evoked motor responses tended to be smaller than normal and, in 7 of 12 patients studies, the reduction in amplitude was associated with prominent and asymmetrical slowing of central motor conduction (16). The most marked findings were in the spinal cord, in which reduction of spinal conduction velocity for the most part correlated with clinical features of corticospinal involvement (Fig. 16-3). The one exception was a patient in whom the plantar response could not be elicited but central motor conduction was demonstrated to be abnormal. In two other instances in which the plantar response was unobtainable, no abnormality was found in central conduction. These results highlight the potential value of the technique for monitoring central pathways in addition to identification of subclinical lesions.

The one reported study of ALS in which magnetic stimulation has been used (18) demonstrated the increased efficacy of this technique over electrical stimulation. Of the 10 patients studied, one-half had clinical evidence of corticospinal involvement. CMCT measurements were found to be abnormal only in those patients with abnormal signs but, in contrast to electrical stimulation studies, reproducible muscle responses were obtained in all cases. The CMCT was twice normal in arm and leg muscles of the most affected case.

COMMENT

The techniques described here for measurement of central and peripheral motor conduction share the advantage of being noninvasive and of providing reliable measures that can be used in sequential studies of the natural history of ALS or in the assessment of possible therapies. They offer the opportunity to examine the biological progression and outcome of the disease process and thus complement the information available from clinical measurements.

REFERENCES

1. Andres PL, Hedlund W, Finison L, Conlon T, Felmus M, Munsat TL. Quantitative motor assessment in amyotrophic lateral sclerosis. *Neurology* 1986; 36;937–41.
2. Appel V, Stewart SS, Smith G, Appel SH. A rating scale for amyotrophic lateral sclerosis: description and preliminary experience. *Ann Neurol* 1987; 22:328–33.
3. Swash M, Ingram D. Preclinical and subclinical events in motor neuron disease. *J Neurol Neurosurg Psychiatry* 1988; 51:165–8.
4. Swash M, Scholtz C, Vowles G, Ingram DA. Selective and asymmetric vulnerability of corticospinal and spinocerebellar tracts in motor neuron disease. *J Neurol Neurosurg Psychiatry* 1988; 51:785–9.
5. Lambert EH. Diagnostic value of electrical stimulation of motor nerves. *Electroencephalogr Clin Neurophysiol* [Suppl] 1962; 22:9–16.
6. Hodes R, Peacock SM Jr, Bodian D. Selective destruction of large motor neurons by poliomyelitis virus, II. *J Neuropathol Exp Neurol* 1949; 8:400-10.
7. Borg J. Conduction velocity and refractory period of single motor nerve fibers in motor neurone disease. *J Neurol Neurosurg Psychiatry* 1984; 47:349–53.

8. Ingram DA, Davis GR, Schwartz MS, Swash M. Motor nerve refractory period and conduction velocity distributions in motor neurone disease. *Electroencephalogr Clin Neurophysiol* 1985; 61:s30.
9. Ingram DA, Davis GR, Swash M. Motor nerve conduction velocity distributions in man: results of a new computer-based collision technique. *Electroencephalogr Clin Neurophysiol* 1987; 66:235–43.
10. Buchthal F, Rosenfalck A. Evoked action potentials and conduction velocity in human sensory nerves. *Brain Res* 1966; 3:1–122.
11. McComas AJ. *Neuromuscular function and disorders*. London: Butterworths, 1977.
12. Stalberg E. Electrophysiological studies of reinnervation in ALS. In: Rowland LP, ed. *Human motor neuron diseases*. New York: Raven Press, 1982.
13. Ingram DA, Davis GR, Swash M. The double collision technique: a new method for measurement of the motor nerve refractory period in man. *Electroencephalogr Clin Neurophysiol* 1987; 66:225–34.
14. Merton PA, Morton HB. Stimulation of the cerebral cortex in the intact human subject. *Nature* 1980; 285:227.
15. Mills KR, Murray NMR. Electrical stimulation over the human vertebral column: which neural elements are excited? *Electroencephalogr Clin Neurophysiol* 1986; 63:582–9.
16. Ingram DA, Swash M. Central motor conduction is abnormal in motor neuron disease. *J Neurol Neurosurg Psychiatry* 1987; 50:159–66.
17. Barker AT, Jalinous R, Freeston IL. Non-invasive stimulation of human motor cortex. *Lancet* 1985; 2:1106–7.
18. Ingram DA. Central motor conduction in neurological disorders: studies with electrical and magnetic brain stimulation. In: Rossini PM, Marsden CD, eds. *Non-invasive stimulation of brain and spinal cord: fundamentals and clinical application*. New York: Liss, 1988: 207–18.
19. Beradelli A, Inghilleri M, Formisano R, Accornero N, Manfredi M. Stimulation of motor tracts in motor neuron disease. *J Neurol Neurosurg Psychiatry* 1987; 50:732–7.

Amyotrophic Lateral Sclerosis,
edited by F. Clifford Rose.
Demos Publications, New York © 1990.

17

The Value of Longitudinal Electromyographic Investigations in Clinical Trials of Motor Neuron Disease

G. H. Wieneke, F. G. I. Jennekens, [1]Y. Van Der Graaf, and P. De Koning

Departments of Neurology and Clinical Neurophysiology, University Hospital, and [1]Department of General Health and Epidemiology, University of Utrecht, Utrecht, The Netherlands

When investigating the influence of drugs on the course of motor neuron disease (MND), two questions need to be answered. The first is whether the drug has any effect at all on the process of degeneration and regeneration of intramuscular nerve fibers in MND. To obtain an answer to this query, a careful investigation of one well-chosen muscle per patient is sufficient. The second question is whether administration of the substance is of advantage to the patients. This second query needs only to be tackled if the answer to the first one is positive and we shall therefore restrict ourselves in the following discussion to the first question.

Melanocortins are related to adrenocorticotropin (ACTH) and α-melanocyte-stimulating hormone (α-MSH). They have been shown to influence regeneration of damaged peripheral nerve fibers (1). The first report on this effect dates from 1980 and since then it has been confirmed and analyzed in a series of studies. The melanocortin moieties of ACTH and α-MSH and a synthetic analog of ACTH4-9 (Org. 2766) enhanced recovery of sensory and motor function after a sciatic nerve crush lesion in the rat. ACTH4-10, α-MSH and Org. 2766 stimulated regeneration of nerve fibers after a crush lesion of the sciatic nerve. The effect is not restricted to myelinated fibers but is also expressed in nonmyelinated fibers, which demonstrates that not only axons of motor neurons but also those of sensory neurons are involved. Besides stimulation of peripheral sprouting, melanocortins also exert beneficial influences on the process of collateral sprouting. There is an enhanced response of intramuscular nerve fibers to the signal, which elicited collateral sprouting and reinnervation in partially denervated soleus muscle of rats treated with Org. 2776 (2).

Of particular interest is the effect of Org. 2766 on cisplatin-induced neuropathy. Cisplatin is a highly effective anti-tumor drug, which is, however, limited in its application by its neurotoxic side-effects. Administration in humans results in a sensory polyneuropathy. In the rat, it has been shown that Org. 2776 counteracts the neurotoxic side-effects of cisplatin without hampering the anti-tumor activity (3,4). Inhibition of nerve toxicity by Org. 2776 also has been observed in experimental diabetic neuropathy and in acrylamide neuropathy (5), which underlines the aspecificity of the effect. It may be assumed that the melanocortin peptides enhance the regenerative power of nerve cells by an as yet unidentified mechanism.

The animal experiments summarized here have laid a sound basis for investigations on the effect of melanocortin peptides on damaged or degenerating nerve fibers in humans and one of the best models is, in our view, MND.

LONGITUDINAL ASSESSMENT OF DEGENERATION AND REGENERATION OF INTRAMUSCULAR NERVE FIBERS

Jitter was chosen as an electromyographic (EMG) variable for the assessment of relatively fast-occurring changes in the process of degeneration and regeneration. Two other variables were chosen for assessment of more long-term changes in muscle innervation: fiber density and motor-unit density. We shall first discuss the rationale for this choice, especially as related to the investigation of the possible beneficial effects of the ACTH4-9 analog Org. 2766 on the process of degeneration and regeneration in MND. Subsequently, we shall present results of a preliminary investigation concerning changes in the EMG variables in patients with MND, within a period of 2–6 months.

Jitter as a rule is increased in muscles from patients with MND; the degree of increase relates to the severity of the disease process (6). The main reason for the increase is probably the presence of regenerating collateral branches of intramuscular nerve fibers, but degenerating still-functioning nerve fibers may also contribute. The effect of Org. 2766 administration on jitter depends on the influence of this drug on the process of degeneration of the motor neurons and on the reinnervation process. Both decrease and increase of jitter are conceivable. Decrease may result from slowing of the degeneration process and from enhanced maturation of regenerated nerve fibers and reinnervated neuromuscular junctions. Temporary increase may be due to acceleration of collateral sprouting and consequently augmentation of the number of immature reinnervated neuromuscular junctions. Increase of the number of reinnervated muscle fibers will be expressed in increase of fiber density.

De Koning et al., in a study on estimation of numbers of motor units in muscle, recently introduced the concept of "motor unit density" (MUD) (7). The term refers to the number of motor units (MUs) in the uptake area of a macro-EMG electrode. The procedure for estimating the MUD is based on a combined registration of single-fiber and macro-EMG and allows for simultaneous registration of jitter, fiber density, and macro-motor-unit potentials (macro-MUP). For a description of the technique of macro-EMG we refer to the original article by Stalberg (8). A macro-MUP represents the temporal and spatial summation of muscle fiber action potentials belonging to one MU. Briefly, the procedure to determine MUD is as follows. A macro-electrode is inserted in one of the large limb muscles 3 cm distal to the endplate zone, and amplitudes and areas of 5 macro-MUPs at different depths in the insertion channel are calculated. In the same insertion channel the supramaximally evoked muscle action potential (macro-SEMAP) is also measured. The ratio of the macro-SEMAP and the mean macro-MUP yields an estimate of the number of motor units in the uptake area of the macro-electrode. The procedure is repeated in three other insertion channels at some distance from each other on a line parallel to the endplate zone. The mean number of MUs at the four insertion channels yields the MUD for that muscle. There is a fairly wide scatter for MUD in the tibialis anterior muscle of controls. MUD decreases ~50% from the 3rd to the 7th decade. Similar results were recently obtained in the musculus biceps branchii by another group using a comparable method (9). In six patients who had progressive spinal muscular atrophy or amyotrophic lateral sclerosis, we found values for the MUD that were well below (50–10%) those of control subjects (7). The areas of the macro-MUPS in these patients were high as is to be expected in a disorder that leads to reinnervation and to enlargement of MUs. If any drug were to slow down the process of degeneration in MND this would cause a slowing of the decrease in MUD.

CHANGES IN ELECTROMYOGRAPHIC VARIABLES IN THE COURSE OF THE DISEASE

To evaluate the changes that occur in time in the chosen EMG variables, we have examined the tibialis anterior muscles of patients with MND. The patients were all ambulant, which allowed them to visit the EMG laboratory. They had little or no bulbar symptoms and no evidence of spasticity. Tendon reflexes were brisk or normal. The tibialis anterior muscle was only slightly weak (Medical Research Council scale: 4+ to 4). The rate of progress of the disease was not very rapid. All patients were willing to cooperate and none of the patients refused for fear of pain to volunteer for a second or a third session.

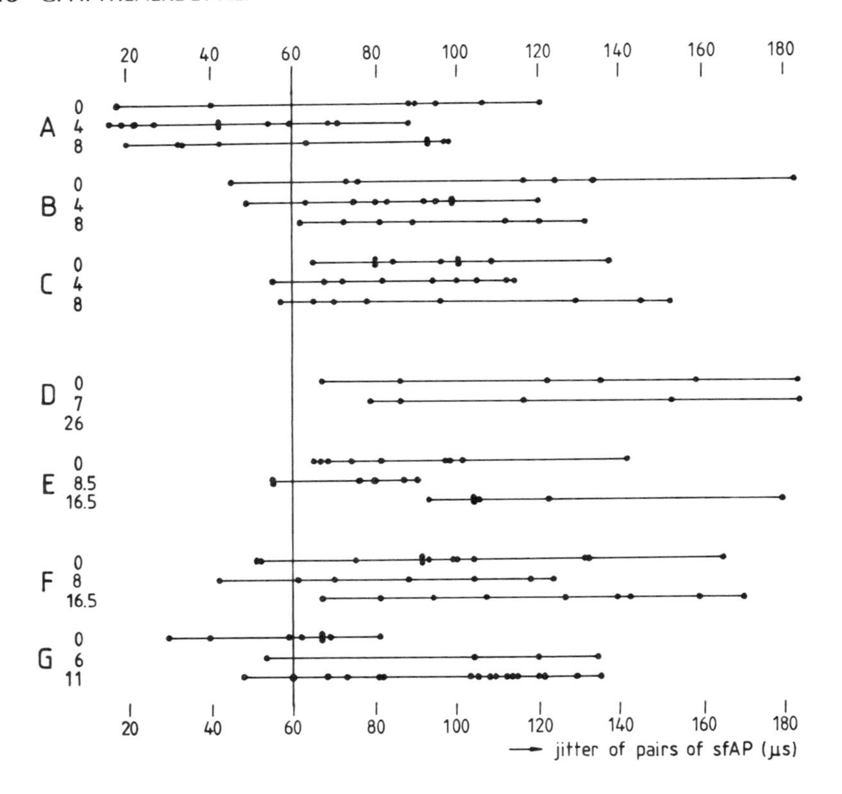

FIG. 17-1. Values for jitter in individual pairs of single-fiber action potentials (SfAP) in seven patients (A–G) with motor neuron disease. Results from three consecutive investigations are represented. The intervals in weeks between the first, second, and third investigations are indicated in the second column. A value of 60 μs is considered to be the upper limit of normal. Reliable jitters in patient D could not be measured during his third investigation.

Intervals between consecutive sessions ranged from 4 to 8 weeks and, exceptionally, 4 months.

Figure 17-1 shows the values for jitters between individual pairs of muscle fibers in the tibialis anterior muscles from seven patients. The range of these jitters was larger than in normal subjects (95% range = 50 μs). Only in some patients were jitters below the normal upper limit of 60 μs found. Patients who showed the most prominent clinical deterioration had the highest jitters. Mean values for jitters were all increased and varied between approximately 60–130 μs (Fig. 17-2). Differences between consecutive investigations in single cases were generally smaller than were differences between patients. Patients A, B, and C were examined with intervals of 4 weeks between subsequent investigations. Analysis of variance of the jitters revealed a significant subject effect ($F = 14.10$, $p < 0.02$), but no significant effect for the repeated investigations

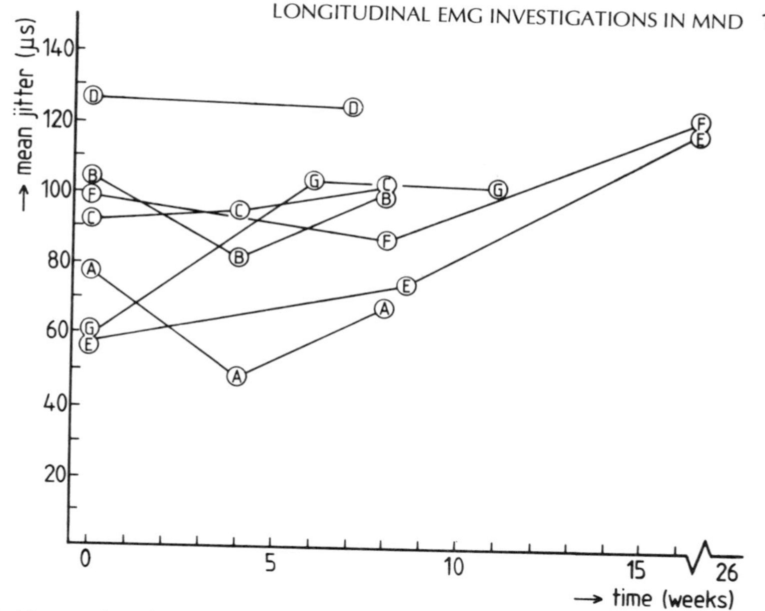

FIG. 17-2. Mean values for jitter measured in three consecutive investigations as function of the time after the first investigation. A–G denote the patients as in Fig. 17-1.

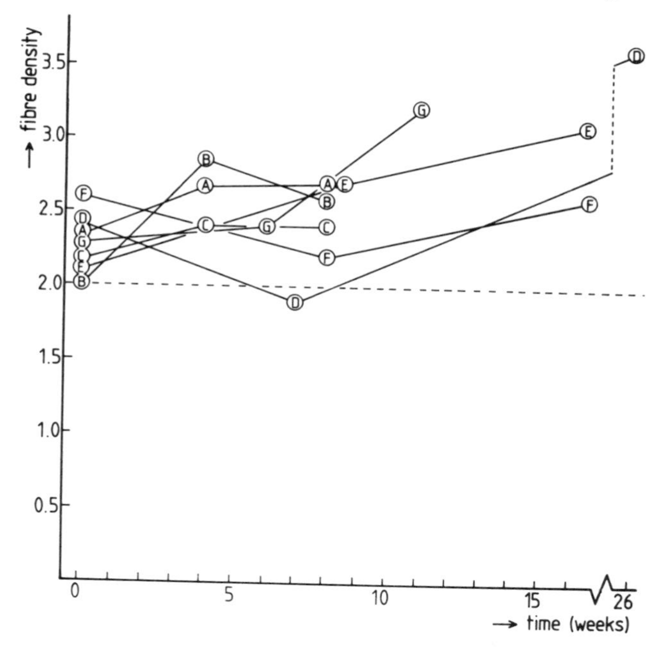

FIG. 17-3. Mean values for fiber density measured in three consecutive investigations as function of the time after the first investigation. A–G denote the patients as in Fig. 17-1.

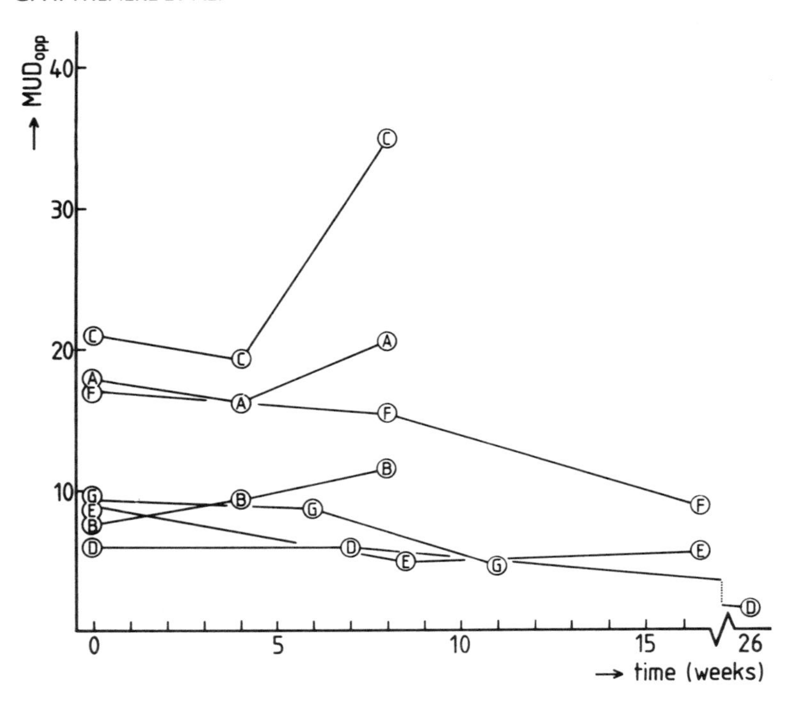

FIG. 17-4. Motor unit densities measured in three consecutive investigations as function of the time after the first investigation. A–G denote the patients as in figure 17-1.

($F = 3.77$, ns). Apparently within a period of 8 weeks the jitter did not change much. In two patients (E, F) who were studied for 16 weeks, a clear increase in mean jitter was found.

Fiber densities mostly exceeded the normal upper limit and varied with a wide scatter from approximately 2 to approximately 3 (Fig 17-3). An analysis of variance in patients examined with 4-week intervals revealed a significant increase of fiber density during the three investigations ($F = 7.23$, $p < 0.05$). A continued increase of fiber density was found in four other patients during a period of 11–26 weeks.

Values for MUD in the patients with MND were generally lower than those in controls. In three patients the values were just low, but in the other cases the values were in the lowest part of the estimated age-dependent distribution of MUD for normals (7). The Z values were -1.9 or lower. The MUD of patients D, E, F, and G showed a decrease in consecutive investigations as is to be expected when fiber density increases (Fig 17-4). The MUD of patients A and B showed a tendency to increase. However, all these effects were within the normal range of variation of the MUD (SD ~25%). Patient C showed a clear increase in the MUD value, which was the result of a very large SEMAP. Additional investigations are required for adequate explanation of this phenomenon.

The results presented here indicate that in the selected category of patients, changes in a period of 4–8 weeks are small for jitter and MUD, and moderate for fiber density (patients A, B, and C). During a longer period the effects of the disease on the electrophysiological variables generally increase (patients D–G).

EXPLANATORY TRIAL WITH EMG VARIABLES

We prefer a multipatient, randomized, double blind, controlled trial to a two-period crossover design (10). Intraindividual differences between predrug and postdrug investigation will be assessed and compared in an experimental and placebo control group. When comparing groups, interindividual differences in jitter, fiber density, and MUD will play a minor role. As shown above, the effect of the natural course of MND on the electrophysiological variables chosen for investigation are small during 4–8 weeks. Thus, when the drug has its effect within 4–8 weeks, the variability in the results due to differences in the rate of progress of the illness between patients will be limited. Changes due to Org. 2776, if present, should be discernible in the electrophysiological variables within a matter of weeks. Histological effects of melanocortin treatment in rat are obvious within days (1). Observations in critically ill patients have shown that humans are able to produce large numbers of collateral sprouts within days (11).

CONCLUSIONS

It is suggested that for the assessment of the effect of drugs in MND in explanatory trials, examination of one skeletal muscle in the patients involved is sufficient. EMG examination may reveal what happens in the process of degeneration and reinnervation in that muscle. We have chosen jitter, fiber density, and MUD as EMG variables. Longitudinal examination of the tibialis anterior muscle in seven patients with moderately progressive MND revealed minor changes in some of these variables within 2 months. Effects if any, of drug remedies should be discernible within this period.

Acknowledgments: The authors are grateful to Mrs. B. Kraan for secretarial assistance and to Mr. H. Veldman for preparing the figures.

REFERENCES

1. De Koning P, Gispen WH. Rationale for the use of melanocortins in neural damage. In: Stein DG, Sabel B, eds. *Pharmalogical approaches to the treatment of brain and spinal cord injuries.* New York: Plenum Press, 1988:253–8.

2. De Koning P, Verhaagen J, Sloot W, et al. Org. 2776 stimulates collateral sprouting in the soleus muscle of the rat following partial denervation. *Muscle Nerve* 1989; 12:353–9.
3. De Koning P, Neyt JP, Jennekens FGI, et al. Org 2776 protects from cisplatin induced neurotoxicity in rats. *Exp Neurol* 1987:1987;746–50.
4. Gerritsen Van der Hoop R, De Koning P, Boven E, et al. Efficacy of the neuropeptide Org. 2776 in the prevention and treatment of cisplatin-induced neurotoxicity in rats. *Eur J Cancer Clin Oncol* 1988;24:637–42.
5. Van Der Zee CEEM, Gerritsen van der Hoop R, Gispen WH. Beneficial effect of ORG2766 in treatment of peripheral neuropathy in streptozocin-induced diabetic rats. *Diabetes* 1989;38:225–30.
6. Stålberg E. Electrophysiological studies of reinnervation in ALS. In: Rowland LP, ed. *Human motor neuron diseases.* New York: Raven Press, 1982:47–59. (Advances in neurology; vol 36.)
7. De Koning P, Wieneke GH, Van Der Most Van Spijk D, et al. Estimation of the number of motor units based on macro-EMG. *J Neurol Neurosurg Psychiatry* 1988;51:403–11.
8. Stålberg E. Macro-EMG, a new recording technique. *J Neurol Neurosurg Psychiatry* 1980;43:475–82.
9. Brown WF, Strong MJ, Snow R. Method for estimating numbers of motor units in biceps branchii muscles and losses of motor units with aging. *Muscle Nerve* 1988;11:423–32.
10. Hills M, Armitage P. The two-period cross-over clinical trial. *Br J Clin Pharm* 1979;8:7–20.
11. Wokke JHJ, Jennekens FGI, van den Oord CJM, et al. Histological investigations of muscle atrophy and endplates in 2 critically ill patients with generalized weakness. *J Neurol Sci* 1988;88:95–106.

Amyotrophic Lateral Sclerosis,
edited by F. Clifford Rose.
Demos Publications, New York © 1990.

18

Critique of Assessment Methodology in Amyotrophic Lateral Sclerosis

Elisabeth S. Louwerse, J. M. B. Vianney de Jong, and [1]Gerald Kuether

Department of Neurology, University of Amsterdam, Academisch Medisch Centrum, Amsterdam, The Netherlands, and [1]Department of Neurology, Technical University of Munich, Neurologische Klinik und Poliklinik, Munich, F.R.G.

Good patient care requires clinical assessments that identify problems, document the natural course of the disease, provide clues for etiopathogenesis, and evaluate therapeutic efficacy. To date, the central and peripheral components of the amyotrophic lateral sclerosis (ALS) motor deficit cannot be measured directly, and there is no generally accepted and straightforward biochemical or physiological measure for the rate of deterioration. Quantitative muscle-strength measurement is probably the most direct assessment of the function of motor neurons, but it cannot alone provide an adequate picture of the patient's life as affected by disease and treatment. For example, when speech and swallowing are deteriorating rapidly, but the limbs are minimally affected, the measurement of muscle strength does not reflect the actual clinical course. Furthermore, what the patient can do with weak muscles is more important than dynamometric values. Especially in ALS, a demeaning disease with a great impact on functional and social well-being, such aspects cannot be overlooked. Bulbar function, activities of daily life, ability of self-care, quality of life, and central motor neuron involvement are as important as they are hard to measure.

REVIEW

Wade et al. (1985) have indicated a number of methodological issues that should be carefully considered in evaluating assessment protocols.

1. *Relevance:* Clinically meaningful and not trivial items should be included but without omitting important variables, the relative importance of which should be reflected in the output score.

2. *Validity:* This means being sure that a test does actually measure whatever it is supposed to measure. In ALS, true validation of assessments is still impossible, because of the lack of a gold standard of its course and the inability of directly measuring the function and number of central and peripheral motor neurons. Validity is therefore estimated by the degree of correlation between test results and other measurements of outcome (criterion-based validity). The test must also have internal consistency, such that all its subsets relate to particular areas of skills or abilities and are not confounded by coassessing clinically separate phenomena.

3. *Reliability:* This is sometimes referred to as repeatability, i.e., if the patient does not change, the score on the test should be the same each time the test is applied whether by the same investigator (intraobserver reliability) or by another investigator (interobserver reliability). Sources of variations are: (a) the patient: effect of training, experience, motivation, verbal coaching, fatigue, age, sex, time of day, concentration, and normal intraindividual changes; (b) the observer: intra- and interobserver variation; (c) the environment: time of day, temperature, humidity, light, noise, and distraction; and (d) the instrument of measurement.

4. *Sensitivity to change:* Each small but clinically meaningful change in the condition of the patient should be reflected equally in the test result.

5. *Quantification:* If possible, accurate, objective, reliable, and sensitive methods should be developed to quantify neurological deficit. However, most clinically important phenomena are not quantitative, but qualitative and can only be recorded in ordinal scales.

6. *Simplicity:* Assessments should be as simple as possible with a proper balance between what is desirable and what is feasible. The amount of discomfort to the patient should be acceptable because, especially in ALS patients, energy and time are limited. The assessment procedure must be easy to learn both for patient and examiner; it should be inexpensive and, if possible, require no specific equipment or room. Simplicity will stimulate widespread use in assessment protocols.

7. *Communicability:* The test result should be easy to understand by all involved in patient care and easy to communicate.

8. *Range:* The range of results should be wide enough to cover the entire spectrum of the measured phenomena in the trial population, with improvement and deterioration receiving equal weight.

9. *Ordinal scales:* Ranks of ordinal scales should be clearly defined, discrete, mutually exclusive, and ordered in hierarchical progression.

10. *Statistical analysis* should be easy.

11. *General acceptance* of the assessment protocol promotes communicability and permits comparison of results from different centers and treatment schedules.

12. *Variables:* The variables recorded depend on the specific purpose of the assessment protocol and the specific question to which it must provide answers.

In ALS, several aspects of the disease may be considered: muscle strength, bulbar function tests, pulmonary function, performance, activities of daily living, ability of self-care, quality of life, and parameters of central and peripheral motor neuron involvement.

To distinguish between these different aspects of ALS, an assessment protocol should not have a single output score, because that will not provide information about the specific condition of the patient.

We thought that it would be useful to tabulate all clinical indexes and quantitative measurements that could be used in ALS, and gather all the information available on their relevance, validity, reliability, and ease in use. On this basis, tentative recommendations can be given on the procedure to use in specific situations, whether in therapeutic trials, diagnosis, prognosis, or as guidelines for symptomatic treatment.

In doing this, three problems had to be confronted. First, most assessment protocols scales are conceived, designed, and used directly in clinical trials without evaluation of their scientific quality. Second, there are at least 230 rating scales for describing impairments of locomotion and 43 for classifying disability and handicap (Feinstein, 1987). Finally, the ideal assessment protocol of ALS does not exist, because it depends on the specific questions asked.

For these reasons, the most important clinical variables will be discussed, as will their relevance, methods of assessment, and the available data on reliability, sensitivity, and validity. In an attempt to identify the most frequently used and generally accepted parameters of disease progression, 26 evaluation protocols (Tables 4 - 21) were studied to advise which methods are best to use.

MUSCLE STRENGTH

In any disease of the motor system, strength is the most direct measure of advancing weakness. Sobue et al. (1983) demonstrated a high correlation between muscle strength before death, and the number of motor neurons after death. However, muscle strength is also influenced by the patient's cooperation, ability to activate motor units, neuromuscular transmission, and efficiency of contraction.

The progression of ALS is most often expressed as the average decrease of muscle strength but it is also important to look at the number of affected muscles or the spread of weakness over the body. When more information becomes available regarding the number of motor neurons needed for the

Table 18-1. *Muscle Strength: Biceps*

MRC grading	0–3				4						5
Percent of normal strength (myometry)	0	10	20	30	40	50	60	70	80	90	100

function of a specific muscle group, loss of strength should be correlated with the number of motor neurons lost. Conradi (personal communication, 1988) has devised a simple and practical map that allows following of the distribution of weakness over time (Fig. 18-1).

Strength may be assessed by manual testing or quantitatively by myometry. In manual muscle-force testing, the force of the muscle is expressed according to the ability to move the limb against the resistance of the examiner, who has to make a judgment based on his or her own experience.

The most widely accepted grading system was devised by the Medical Research Council (MRC) and consists of six categories (0–5). Category 4 (moving against resistance) is too broad; for example, the biceps may lose 97% of its strength before the score changes from 4 to 3 (Table 18-1).

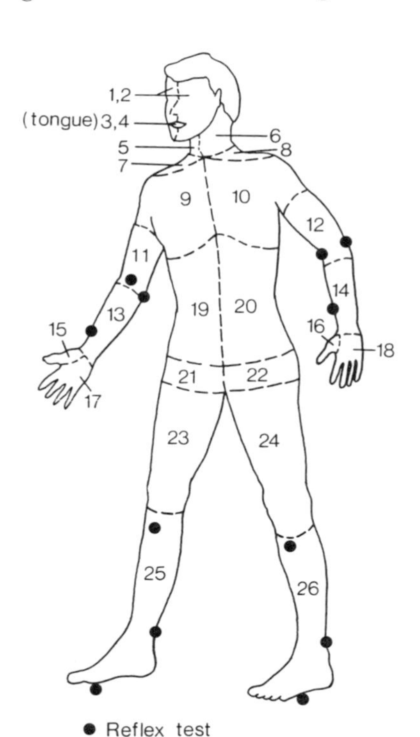

FIG. 18-1. Follow-up of the topographic distribution of weakness, atrophy, and reflex abnormalities is facilitated by this diagram, devised by S. Conradi (reprinted with permission).

Table 18-2. *Advantages and Disadvantages of Manual Muscle Strength Testing Versus Myometry*

Manual muscle strength testing	Myometry
Qualitative	Quantitative
Produces disproportionate ordinal data, not permitting addition of scores, but analysis of frequencies only	Produces interval data
Limited number of grades, poor sensitivity for change, especially at the upper range of strength	Sensitive to change
Also measures very weak muscles	Only capable of measuring strength when the muscle is able to build up force against resistance (floor effect)
Widely used in general practice	Used by only a few investigators
Communicable	Not communicable to all clinicians
Quick	Time consuming
Patient friendly	Patient burden considerable
Easy	Instruction and experience of the investigator required
Also suitable for obese and spastic patients	Positioning difficult; inaccurate measurement of spastic and obese patients
Subjective assessment (propriocepsis of the investigator)	Objective assessment
Assessment influenced by the weight of the limb and the strength of the investigator	Assessment in isokinetic myometry influenced by limb weight
Good test–retest reliability	Good test–retest reliability

In addition, the percentage of normal force required to move the limb against gravity varies from 1 to more than 30% for different muscle groups (Beasly, 1961).

The MRC grading system has the disadvantage of being insensitive at the upper range of strength and producing disproportionate ordinal data, which permit analysis of frequencies but not the addition of scores.

Strength is measured quantitatively by myometry which has both advantages and disadvantages relative to manual muscle-strength testing (Table 18-2).

Quantitative strength measurement can be performed under either isometric or isokinetic conditions. In isokinetic testing, the torque produced by a muscle group is recorded as the limb moves through the entire range of motion with a preset speed. The worst disadvantage of the isokinetic method is that variables such as muscle length, velocity of movement, and limb weight affect the measurement. In addition, the equipment is expensive and the

Table 18-3. *Advantages and Disadvantages of Hand-Held Versus Strain-Gauge Myometers*

Hand-held myometer	Strain-gauge myometer
Maximal measurable strength is limited by the maximal strength of the investigator; method not suitable for measuring minor degrees of weakness in adults (ceiling effect)	Also very strong muscles may be tested (up to 100 kg)
Rather inexpensive	More expensive
Pocket format	Special table or chair required
Portable, can possibly be used at home-visits and in the ward	Not portable, patient has to be transported to a specially equipped room
Patient-friendly	Less patient-friendly

procedure laborious. For these reasons, in most ALS protocols strength is usually measured under isometric conditions, i.e., the examiner resists movement of the muscle group under study and holds the limb immobile. In positioning, the influence of gravity has to be minimized to allow testing of very weak muscles and also because the effect of gravity varies for each muscle group and with limb weight.

For quantitative isometric strength measurement, different types of myometers are available: spring balances, cable tensiometers, strain gauges, and hand-held myometers. In ALS research, strain gauges and hand-held myometers are most frequently used (Table 18-3). Using strain gauges, the patient pulls against an immovable strap, and is asked to build up as much force as possible. With use of a hand-held myometer, the instrument is interposed between examiner and patient; when the examiner overcomes the patient's contraction, the force is recorded. Both myometers have their specific advantages and disadvantages.

Test–retest reliability is good for both methods (Wiles and Karni, 1983; van der Ploeg and Oosterhuis, 1984; Andres et al., 1986) with a test–retest correlation $r = 0.90$. The normal individual variation of muscle strength in patients is probably responsible for the major part of the variation. Reproducibility of measurement is increased by exactly defined positioning of patient and limb part, by accurate stabilization of proximal joints, and by invariable positioning of myometer or strap, standardized muscle contraction–relaxation time, instruction of the patient, and verbal encouragement (Smidt and Rogers, 1982; de Boer et al., 1982; Van der Ploeg and Oosterhuis, 1984).

To reduce data and improve clinical relevance, quantitative strength measurements, expressed in kilograms or newtons, should be compared with sex-, age-, height-, and weight-matched controls and be expressed as a percentage of normal. At present no adequate bank of such data is available.

Table 18-4. *Components of Evaluation-Protocols*

Author	Year	Pulmonary function	Bulbar function	Muscle force	Timed motor functions	Performance	ADL functions	Dependency	Course of EMG
Norris	1974	+	+	+	−	−	+	−	−
Rivera	1980	+	+	+	−	+	+	−	+
Brooke	1981	+	+	+	+	+	+	+	−
Engel	1983	+	+	+	−	−	−	−	−
Bradley	1984	+	+	+	+	+	+	−	+
Gracco	1984	−	+	+	−	−	−	−	−
Newrick	1984	−	−	−	−	−	+	+	−
Saida	1984	+	+	+	+	+	+	−	−
Sufit	1984	+	−	+	+	+	+	+	−
Andres	1986	+	+	+	+	−	−	−	−
Brooke	1986	+	+	+	+	−	−	−	+
Caroscio	1986	+	+	+	+	+	−	−	−
Dalakas	1986	+	+	+	−	−	+	−	−
Mitumoto	1986	+	+	+	+	+	+	+	+
Appel	1987	+	+	+	+	+	+	−	−
Brooks	1987	+	+	+	+	+	+	−	−
Guiloff	1987	+	+	+	+	−	+	−	−
Kuether	1987	+	+	+	−	−	+	−	+
Sinaki	1987	−	−	+	−	+	+	−	−
Thielen	1987	+	+	+	−	−	+	−	−
Hillel	1988	−	+	−	−	+	+	+	−
Honda	1988	+	−	−	−	−	+	−	−
Iwata	1988	+	+	−	−	+	+	+	−
Jerusalem	1988	+	+	+	+	+	+	−	−
Pinelli	1988	−	−	+	+	−	−	−	+
Plaitakis	1988	−	+	+	−	+	+	−	−
Total	26	20	21	22	13	14	20	6	6

ADL, activities of daily living; EMG, electromyography

Muscle strength was assessed in 22 of the 26 protocols (Table 18-4)—manual muscle strength testing in 9 studies, dynamometry in 7 studies, both methods in 3 studies, and method unspecified in 3 protocols (Table 18-5).

In most ALS protocols a variety of muscle groups in the arms, trunk, and legs are tested bilaterally (Tables 18-6–9). The number of muscles tested varies from 6 to 58 (average of 27.7). A standardized selection of muscles has not been generally agreed, being selected either on the basis of the number of motor neurons involved, their predilection for being affected by the disease, the reliability of measurements, or their value for activities of daily life.

Table 18-5. *Muscle Strength Testing*

						Technique Used			
		Body part			Total no. of muscle groups tested	Manual muscle force tests	Myometry		
Author	Year	Arms	Trunk	Legs			Hand-held	Strain gauge	Grip Str.
Norris	1974	Muscles unspecified			58	+	–	–	–
Rivera	1980	Muscles unspecified			26	+	–	–	–
Brooke	1981	+	–	+	34	+	–	–	–
Engel	1983	Muscles unspecified			?	Technique unspecified			
Bradley	1984	Muscles unspecified			36	–	–	+	+
Gracco	1984	Muscles unspecified			?	–	–	+	–
Newrick	1984	–	–	–	–	–	–	–	–
Saida	1984	Muscles unspecified			?	Technique unspecified			
Sufit	1984	+	–	+	34	+	–	–	+
Andres	1986	+	–	+	20	–	–	+	+
Brooke	1986	+	–	+	36	+	–	–	+
Caroscio	1986	+	–	+	28	+	+	–	+
Dalakas	1986	Muscles unspecified			22	+	–	–	–
Mitsumoto	1986	+	+	+	30	+	–	+	+
Appel	1987	+	–	+	32	+	–	–	+
Brooks	1987	+	–	–	8	–	"Myometry"		
Guiloff	1987	+	–	+	8	–	+	–	–
Kuether	1987	+	+	+	46	+	–	+	+
Sinaki	1987	Muscle unspecified			?	Technique unspecified			
Thielen	1987	Muscles unspecified			?	+	–	–	–
Hillel	1988	–	–	–	–	–	–	–	–
Honda	1988	–	–	–	–	–	–	–	–
Iwata	1988	–	–	–	–	–	–	–	–
Jerusalem	1988	+	–	+	20	–	–	+	+
Pinelli	1988	–	–	+	6–8	–	–	+	–
Plaitakis	1988	+	–	+	26	+	–	–	–
Total	26	12	2	12	6–58	12	2	7	10

BULBAR FUNCTION

Although essential functions as speech and swallowing are frequently affected in ALS, the scientific quality of the assessment of these symptoms has received little attention. In most ALS protocols bulbar functions are rated (Table 18-10) without evaluation of reliability or validity of the assessment.

Quantitative measurements of bulbar function are not easy. Maximal voluntary contraction of lips, jaw, and tongue can be assessed by specially designed

Table 18-6. *Muscle Groups of Arm Tested*

Author	Year	Arm	Hand							
		Elbow flex.	Elbow ext.	Wrist flex.	Wrist ext.	Finger flex.	Finger ext.	Finger Ab-duct.	Lat. pinch.	Grip force
Norris	1974		Muscle groups not specified							
Rivera	1980		Muscle groups not specified							
Brooke	1981	+	+	+	+					
Engel	1983		Muscle groups not specified							
Bradley	1984		Muscle groups not specified							
Gracco	1984		Muscle groups not specified							
Newrick	1984									
Saida	1984		Muscle groups not specified							
Sufit	1984	+	+	+	+					
Andres	1986	+	+	+						+
Brooke	1986	+	+	+	+	+	+	+		+
Caroscio	1986	+	+	+	+	+	+			+
Dalakas	1986		Muscle groups not specified							
Mitsumoto	1986	+	+	+	+					+
Appel	1987	+	+	+	+	+	+		+	
Brooks	1987			+	+	+				
Guiloff	1987		+				+			
Kuether	1987	+	+	+	+	+	+	+		+
Sinaki	1987		Muscle groups not specified							
Thielen	1987		Muscle groups not specified							
Hillel	1988									
Honda	1988									
Iwata	1988									
Jerusalem	1988	+	+		+					+
Pinelli	1988									
Plaitakis	1988	+	+	+	+	+	+	+		
Total	26	10	11	10	10	6	6	3	1	7

force transducers (Barlow and Abbs, 1984), but not the strength and function of pharyngeal and larygeal muscles. Diadochokinetic speech rate and timed drinking and eating provide interval data but, in later stages of the disease, the ability to complete these tasks is often lost and test results do not directly reflect the actual function of bulbar muscles in daily life. This means that, in addition to timed bulbar function tests, subjective ratings of intelligibility of speech, chewing, swallowing, drooling, and emotional control need to be obtained. An easily administered, valid, and reliable index of bulbar functions is the Frenchay Dysarthria Assessment (Enderby, 1983).

Table 18-7. *Muscle Groups Trunk and Shoulder Girdle Tested*

		Trunk					Shoulder			
Author	Year	Neck-flex.	Neck-ext.	Neck-rot.	Trunk-flex.	Trunk-ext.	Sh. abd.	Sh. flex.	Sh. ext.	Sh. exrot.
Norris	1974	Muscle groups unspecified					Muscle groups unspecified			
Rivera	1980	Muscle groups unspecified					Muscle groups unspecified			
Brooke	1981	+	+	–	–	–	+	–	–	+
Engel	1983	Muscle groups unspecified					Muscle groups unspecified			
Bradley	1984	Muscle groups unspecified					Muscle groups unspecified			
Gracco	1984	Muscle groups unspecified					Muscle groups unspecified			
Newrick	1984	–	–	–	–	–	–	–	–	–
Saida	1984	Muscle groups unspecified					Muscle groups unspecified			
Sufit	1984	+	+	–	–	–	+	–	–	+
Andres	1986	–	–	–	–	–	–	+	+	–
Brooke	1986	–	–	–	–	–	+	–	–	–
Caroscio	1986	–	–	–	–	–	+	–	–	–
Dalakas	1986	Muscle groups unspecified					Muscle groups unspecified			
Mitsumoto	1986	+	+	–	–	–	+	–	–	–
Appel	1987	–	–	–	–	–	+	–	–	–
Brooks	1987	–	–	–	–	–	–	–	–	–
Guiloff	1987	–	–	–	–	–	+	–	–	–
Kuether	1987	+	+	+	–	–	+	–	–	–
Sinaki	1987	Muscle groups unspecified					Muscle groups unspecified			
Thielen	1987	Muscle groups unspecified					Muscle groups unspecified			
Hillel	1988	–	–	–	–	–	–	–	–	–
Honda	1988	–	–	–	–	–	–	–	–	–
Iwata	1988	–	–	–	–	–	–	–	–	–
Jerusalem	1988	–	–	–	–	–	–	+	+	–
Pinelli	1988	–	–	–	–	–	–	–	–	–
Plaitakas	1988	–	–	–	–	–	+	–	–	–
Total	26	4	4	1	0	0	9	2	2	2

PULMONARY FUNCTION

Patients with ALS usually die from respiratory problems. Respiratory function is not only one of the most important predictors of survival, but also a major determinant of functional capability, because decreased ventilation limits exercise capacity.

In ALS research, maximal voluntary ventilation (Fallat et al, 1979) and maximal inspiratory and expiratory pressure (Griggs et al., 1981) may be sensitive parameters. In some patients, the earliest indicators of respiratory involvement are a high residual volume and dyscoordination of expiratory effort. The maximum expiratory pressure is of greatest predictive value in assessing the need for tracheostomy (Cohen et al., 1985).

Table 18-8. *Muscle Groups of Thighs and Pelvic Girdle Tested*

Author	Year	Hip flex.	Hip ext.	Hip abd.	Knee flex.	Knee ext.
Norris	1974		Muscle groups not specified			
Rivera	1980		Muscle groups not specified			
Brooke	1981	+	+	+	+	+
Engel	1983		Muscle groups not specified			
Bradley	1984		Muscle groups not specified			
Gracco	1984		Muscle groups not specified			
Newrick	1984	–	–	–	–	–
Saida	1984		Muscle groups not specified			
Sufit	1984	+	+	+	+	+
Andres	1986	+	+	–	+	+
Brooke	1986	+	+	+	+	+
Caroscio	1986	+	–	–	+	+
Dalakas	1986		Muscle groups not specified			
Mitsumoto	1986	+	+	–	+	+
Appel	1987	+	–	–	+	+
Brooks	1987	–	–	–	–	–
Guiloff	1987	+	–	–	–	–
Kuether	1987	+	–	+	+	+
Sinaki	1987		Muscle groups not specified			
Thielen	1987		Muscle groups not specified			
Hillel	1988	–	–	–	–	–
Honda	1988	–	–	–	–	–
Iwata	1988	–	–	–	–	–
Jerusalem	1988	+	+	–	+	+
Pinelli	1988	–	–	–	–	+
Plaitakis	1988	+	–	–	+	+
Total	26	11	6	4	10	11

Pulmonary function was assessed in 20 of the 26 study protocols (Table 18-4), the most frequently used being forced vital capacity and maximum voluntary ventilation (Table 18-11). Whichever tests are chosen, pulmonary function must always be expressed as percentage of normal, because it varies with age, sex, height, and weight.

PERFORMANCE TESTS

Performance tests reflect ability of the patient to function in daily life better than muscle strength measurements do, but are subject to environmental, physical, and emotional influences, and rehabilitation and aids. As a consequence, they provide a very indirect, inaccurate measurement of motor neuron function. In Duchenne muscular dystrophy, myometry and percent MRC score

Table 18-9. *Muscle Groups of Leg and Foot Tested*

		Foot					
Author	Year	Plant. flex.	Dorsi-flex.	Inverters	Everters	Toe—flex.	Toe—ext.
Norris	1974			Muscle groups not specified			
Rivera	1980			Muscle groups not specified			
Brooke	1981	+	+	+	+	–	–
Engel	1983			Muscle groups not specified			
Bradley	1984			Muscle groups not specified			
Gracco	1984			Muscle groups not specified			
Newrick	1984	–	–	–	–	–	–
Saida	1984			Muscle groups not specified			
Sufit	1984	+	+	+	+	–	–
Andres	1986	–	+	–	–	–	–
Brooke	1986	+	+	–	+	–	–
Caroscio	1986	+	+	–	–	–	–
Dalakas	1986			Muscle groups not specified			
Mitsumoto	1986	–	–	–	+	+	–
Appel	1987	+	+	–	–	+	+
Brooks	1987	–	–	–	–	–	–
Guiloff	1987	–	–	–	–	–	–
Kuether	1987	+	+	+	+	–	–
Sinaki	1987			Muscle groups not specified			
Thielen	1987			Muscle groups not specified			
Hillel	1988	–	–	–	–	–	–
Honda	1988	–	–	–	–	–	–
Iwata	1988	–	–	–	–	–	–
Jerusalem	1988	–	+	–	–	–	–
Pinelli	1988	–	+	–	–	–	+
Plaitakis	1988	+	+	–	–	–	–
Total	26	7	10	3	5	2	2

have a greater statistical power in therapeutic trials than do walking times, interval to loss of ambulation, or motor ability tests (Dubowitz et al., 1986). The explanation may be that these parameters do not change continuously in time, as does muscle strength, but at intervals that depend on critical levels of motor function and on environmental factors. This explains why the relationship between muscle strength measurements and performance tests is not linear (Andres et al., 1987); both give important information regarding the patient, but not the same information.

To date there is no agreed standard tests for testing motor function in ALS, but the most frequently used are shown in Tables 18-12 and 18-13.

Table 18-10. *Bulbar Function*

Author	Year	Grading of function				Timed functions			Muscle force	
		Speech	Chewing	Swallowing	Emot. Contr.	Speech Rate	Eating	Drinking	Myometry	Grading
Norris	1974	+	+	+	+	–	–	–	–	–
Rivera	1980	+	–	+	–	–	–	–	–	–
Brooke	1981	–	–	–	–	–	–	–	–	–
Engel	1983	+	–	–	–	–	–	–	Techn. unspec.	
Bradley	1984	+	–	+	–	+	–	+	–	+
Gracco	1984	–	–	–	–	–	–	–	+	–
Newrick	1984	+	+	+	–	–	–	–	–	–
Saida	1984	+	+	+	+	+	–	+	–	–
Sufit	1984	–	–	–	–	–	–	–	–	–
Andres	1986	–	–	–	–	+	–	–	–	–
Brooke	1986	–	–	–	–	+	–	+	–	–
Caroscio	1986	+	–	+	–	+	–	–	–	+
Dalakas	1986	+	+	+	+	–	–	–	–	–
Mitsumoto	1986	+	+	+	–	+	–	+	–	–
Appel	1987	+	–	+	–	–	–	–	–	–
Brooks	1987	+	+	+	+	+	–	–	+	–
Guiloff	1987	+	+	+	+	–	–	+	–	+
Kuether	1987	+	+	+	+	–	–	–	–	–
Sinaki	1987	–	–	–	–	–	–	–	–	–
Thielen	1987	+	+	+	+	–	–	–	–	–
Hillel	1988	+	–	+	–	–	–	–	–	–
Honda	1988	–	–	–	–	–	–	–	–	–
Iwata	1988	+	+	+	–	–	–	–	–	–
Jerusalem	1988	+	–	–	–	+	+	+	–	+
Pinelli	1988	–	–	–	–	–	–	–	–	–
Plaitakis	1988	+	+	+	–	–	–	–	–	+
Total	26	18	11	16	7	9	1	6	2	5

TIMED MOTOR ACTIVITIES

In timed motor activities tests, the patient is asked to perform a certain task as fast as possible. The advantage of timed activities is that interval data are produced that facilitate statistical analysis and that are more sensitive to change than such ordinal data as disability scales or performance tests. Frequently used tests in ALS research are timed walk, climbing and descending stairs, rising from a chair, or from lying supine, and the peg board test (Tables 18-14 and 15).

Table 18-11. *Pulmonary Function*

Author	Year	Forced vital cap.	Max volunt. vent.	Max exp. press.	Max insp. press.	Peak exp. flow	Minute ventil. at max. work	Resp. rate	Dyspnea	Cough force
Norris	1974	+	+	–	–	–	–	–	+	+
Rivera	1980	+	–	+	–	–	–	–	–	–
Brooke	1981	+	+	+	–	–	–	–	–	–
Engel	1983	+	–	–	–	–	–	–	–	+
Bradley	1984	+	+	–	–	–	–	–	+	+
Gracco	1984	–	–	–	–	–	–	–	–	–
Newrick	1984	–	–	–	–	–	–	–	–	–
Saida	1984	+	–	–	–	–	+	–	+	+
Sufit	1984	+	+	–	+	–	–	–	–	–
Andres	1986	+	+	–	–	–	–	–	–	–
Brooke	1986	+	+	+	–	–	–	–	–	–
Caroscio	1986	+	–	–	–	–	–	–	+	–
Dalakas	1986	+	–	–	–	–	–	–	–	+
Mitsumoto	1986	+	–	–	+	–	–	+	–	–
Appel	1987	+	–	–	–	–	–	–	–	–
Brooks	1987	+	+	–	–	–	–	–	+	+
Guiloff	1987	+	–	+	+	+	–	–	+	+
Kuether	1987	+	–	–	–	–	–	–	+	+
Sinaki	1987	–	–	–	–	–	–	–	–	–
Thielen	1987	+	–	–	–	–	–	–	+	+
Hillel	1988	–	–	–	–	–	–	–	–	–
Honda	1988	–	–	–	–	–	–	–	+	–
Iwata	1988	–	–	–	–	–	–	–	+	–
Jerusalem	1988	+	+	–	–	–	–	–	–	+
Pinelli	1988	–	–	–	–	–	–	–	–	–
Plaitakis	1988	–	–	–	–	–	–	–	–	–
Total	26	18	8	4	3	1	1	1	10	10

EXERCISE-CAPACITY TESTS

Sanjak et al. (1987) showed that ALS patients have smaller work capacity and require more oxygen than normal controls. Both in planning a rehabilitation program and in testing new drugs, exercise capacity tests may prove useful. Maximal aerobic exercise capacity may be measured by bicycle ergometry (Sanguq et al., 1984; Sanjak et al, 1987). Although fatigue is one of the most disabling symptoms in ALS, the quantification of endurance has received little attention and in only 3 of the 26 protocols studied was exercise capacity or fatigability of muscle strength measured (Sufit et al., 1984; Brooks et al., 1987; Guiloff and Eckland, 1987).

Table 18-12. *Performance Tests (Not Timed) of the Arms*

Author	Year	Raise arms	Hand function
Norris	1974	–	–
Rivera	1980	–	–
Brooke	1981	+	+
Engel	1983	–	–
Bradley	1984	Not specified	
Gracco	1984	–	–
Newrick	1984	–	–
Saida	1984	–	–
Sufit	1984	+	+
Andres	1986	–	–
Brooke	1986	–	–
Caroscio	1986	–	–
Dalakas	1986	–	–
Mitsumoto	1986	+	–
Appel	1987	+	+
Brooks	1987	+	+
Guiloff	1987	–	–
Kuether	1987	–	–
Sinaki	1987	+	–
Thielen	1987	–	–
Hillel	1988	–	–
Honda	1988	–	–
Iwata	1988	+	+
Jerusalem	1988	+	–
Pinelli	1988	–	–
Plaitakis	1988	–	–
Total		8	5

ACTIVITIES OF DAILY LIVING

In disability scales, activities of daily life (ADL) evaluated can be divided into (a) self care; (b) physical activities; and (c) role activities, social and at work.

Most ADL scales assess activities such as dressing, grooming, bathing, managing the toilet, walking, managing stairs, transferring from bed to chair, feeding and continence. Social activities, such as going to a concert, shopping, and visiting, which are very important for the quality of life, are not assessed.

What people *can* manage may not be what they actually *do* (Andrews and Stewart, 1979). Because disability scales must give an impression about the patient's actual functioning in daily life, it is clinically more relevant to assess what the patient actually *does*.

Table 18-13. *Performance Tests (Not Timed) of Trunk and Legs*

Author	Year	Rise from supine	Roll over in bed	Walk	Stand	Stand on heels & toes	Rise from chair	Rise from floor	Raise legs
Norris	1974	–	–	–	–	–	–	–	–
Rivera	1980	–	–	–	–	–	–	–	–
Brooke	1981	–	–	+	–	–	–	–	–
Engel	1983	–	–	–	–	–	–	–	–
Bradley	1984	ADL activities, not specified							
Gracco	1984	–	–	–	–	–	–	–	–
Newrick	1984	–	–	–	–	–	–	–	–
Saida	1984	–	–	–	–	–	–	–	–
Sufit	1984	–	–	+	–	–	–	–	–
Andres	1986	–	–	–	–	–	–	–	–
Brooke	1986	–	–	–	–	–	–	–	–
Caroscio	1986	–	–	+	–	–	–	–	–
Dalakas	1986	–	–	–	–	–	–	–	–
Mitsumoto	1986	+	+	–	–	–	–	–	+
Appel	1987	–	–	–	–	–	–	–	–
Brooks	1987	–	–	+	–	–	–	–	–
Guiloff	1987	–	–	–	–	–	–	–	–
Kuether	1987	–	–	–	–	–	–	–	–
Sinaki	1987	–	–	–	–	–	–	–	–
Thielen	1987	–	–	–	–	–	–	–	–
Hillel	1988	–	–	–	–	–	–	–	–
Honda	1988	–	–	–	–	–	–	–	–
Iwata	1988	+	–	–	–	–	–	–	–
Jerusalem	1988	+	–	–	+	+	+	+	–
Pinelli	1988	–	–	+	–	–	–	–	–
Plaitakis	1988	–	–	+	–	–	–	–	–
Total	26	3	1	6	1	1	1	1	1

The literature abounds with disability scales and Donaldson et al. (1973) has reviewed 25 of them. Although they do mutually correlate to a high degree, no single one has yet generally been accepted. Most ADL scales lack sensitivity to change at the upper range of maximal disability (Skilbeck et al., 1983). In neurology, the Barthel Index (Mahoney and Barthel, 1965) is one of the best known, and is used extensively in cerebrovascular disorders. The scale is simple and quick to complete. Ten daily activities are assessed: feeding, going to the toilet, bathing, grooming, dressing, bed–chair transfer, mobility, managing stairs, and bladder and bowel control. The validity of the Barthel Index in stroke patients is good (Wylie and White, 1964; Gresham et al., 1980; Wade and Langton Hewer, 1987) because it correlates well with other measurements of outcome and functional capacity such as the Katz Index (Katz et al., 1963) and Kenny self-care

Table 18-14. *Timed Motor Function Tests of the Arms*

Author	Year	Peg board	Dial a phone number	Put on shirt	Cut out square	Cut theraplast	Propel Wheel chair	Close & open safety pin	Place blocks	Rotate stick
Norris	1974	–	–	–	–	–	–	–	–	–
Rivera	1980	–	–	–	–	–	–	–	–	–
Brooke	1981	–	–	+	+	–	+	–	–	–
Engel	1983	–	–		–	–	–	–	–	–
Bradley	1984				Tests not specified					
Gracco	1984	–	–	–	–	–	–	–	–	–
Newrick	1984	–	–	–	–	–	–	–	–	–
Saida	1984	–	–	+	–	–	–	–	–	–
Sufit	1984	–	–	+	+	–	+	–	–	–
Andres	1986	+	+	–	–	–	–	–	–	–
Brooke	1986	–	–	–	–	–	–	+	–	–
Caroscio	1986	–	–	–	–	–	–	–	–	–
Dalakas	1986	–	–	–	–	–	–	–	–	–
Mitsumoto	1986	–	–	–	–	–	–	–	–	–
Appel	1987	+	–	–	–	+	+	–	+	–
Brooks	1987	+	+	–	–	–	–	–	–	–
Guiloff	1987	–	–	–	–	–	–	–	–	–
Kuether	1987	–	–	–	–	–	–	–	–	–
Sinaki	1987	–	–	–	–	–	–	–	–	–
Thielen	1987	–	–	–	–	–	–	–	–	–
Hillel	1988	–	–	–	–	–	–	–	–	–
Honda	1988	–	–	–	–	–	–	–	–	–
Iwata	1988	–	–	–	–	–	–	–	–	–
Jerusalem	1988	+	–	–	–	–	–	–	–	+
Pinelli	1988	–	–	–	–	–	–	–	–	–
Plaitakis	1988	–	–	–	–	–	–	–	–	–
Total	26	4	2	3	2	1	3	1	1	1

evaluation (Donaldson et al., 1973). Of these three, the Barthel Index has the advantages of completeness, popularity, sensitivity to change and ease in use, but no results of test–retest reliability have yet been reported.

In ALS, unlike stroke, disability scales are seldom used, even though good ones are essential in staging the disease and identifying the patient's day-to-day problems. An adequate scale will have consequences for timely symptomatic care. In addition, the loss of some functional ability may prove to have prognostic value, as Wade and Langton Hewer (1987) have demonstrated in stroke patients.

Despite the lack of a generally accepted ADL scale, various functional abilities are evaluated in ALS assessment protocols (Tables 18-16 and 18-17), but without the quality of the grading systems having been ascertained.

Table 18-15. *Timed Motor Function Tests of Trunk and Legs*

Author	Year	Walk	Stairs up & down	Step onto foot stool	Step onto chair	Rise from chair	Rise from floor	Raise head	Rise from supine
Norris	1974	–	–	–	–	–	–	–	–
Rivera	1980	–	–	–	–	–	–	–	–
Brooke	1981	+	+	+	–	+	–	–	+
Engel	1983	–	–	–	–	–	–	–	–
Bradley	1984			Three tests, not specified					
Gracco	1984	–	–	–	–	–	–	–	–
Newrick	1984	–	–	–	–	–	–	–	–
Saida	1984	+	+	–	–	–	–	–	–
Sufit	1984	+	+	–	–	+	–	–	+
Andres	1986	+	–	–	–	–	–	–	–
Brooke	1986	+	+	+	+	+	+	–	–
Caroscio	1986	+	–	–	–	–	–	–	–
Dalakas	1986	–	–	–	–	–	–	–	–
Mitsumoto	1986	+	–	–	–	+	–	–	–
Appel	1987	+	+	–	–	+	–	–	+
Brooks	1987	+	–	+	–	+	+	–	–
Guiloff	1987	+	–	–	–	–	–	–	–
Kuether	1987	–	–	–	–	–	–	–	–
Sinaki	1987	–	–	–	–	–	–	–	–
Thielen	1987	–	–	–	–	–	–	–	–
Hillel	1988	–	–	–	–	–	–	–	–
Honda	1988	–	–	–	–	–	–	–	–
Iwata	1988	–	–	–	–	–	–	–	–
Jerusalem	1988	+	–	–	–	–	–	+	–
Pinelli	1988	+	–	–	–	–	–	–	–
Plaitakis	1988	–	–	–	–	–	–	–	–
Total	26	12	5	3	1	6	2	1	3

HANDICAP INDICES

ADL scales, in which a variety of daily activities are evaluated, differ from handicap scales, in which the patient's overall function, ability of self-care and dependency on help are recorded. Handicap scales indicate to what extent patients can look after themselves, but this ability of self-care has been assessed in only 2 of the 26 evaluation protocols (18-18).

The Karnofsky Performance Status Index assesses the patient's independence and symptom level (Karnofsky and Burchenall, 1949) and is widely used in cancer research. Its validity is good (Mor et al., 1984; Schag et al., 1984) and its reliability can be improved by clearly defining each performance level

Table 18-16. *Activities of Daily Living—I*

Author	Year	Walk	Manage stairs	Manage toilet	Bed–chair transfer	Bed activity	Bath	Dress	Groom
Norris	1974	+	+	–	+	+	–	+	–
Rivera	1980	+	+	Other ADL activities, not specified					
Brooke	1981	+	+	–	–	–	–	–	–
Engel	1983	–	–	–	–	–	–	–	–
Bradley	1984			ADL activites, not specified					
Gracco	1984	–	–	–	–	–	–	–	–
Newrick	1984	+	+	+	+	–	+	+	+
Saida	1984	+	+	–	+	+	–	+	–
Sufit	1984	+	+	–	–	–	–	–	–
Andres	1986	timed	–	–	–	–	–	–	–
Brooke	1986	timed	–	–	–	–	–	–	–
Caroscio	1986	timed	–	–	–	–	–	–	–
Dalakas	1986	+	+	–	+	+	–	+	–
Mitsumoto	1986	+	–	–	–	+	–	–	+
Appel	1987	+	+	–	–	–	–	+	–
Brooks	1987	+	+	–	+	+	–	+	–
Guiloff	1987	+	+	–	+	+	–	+	–
Kuether	1987	+	+	–	+	+	–	+	–
Sinaki	1987	+	+	–	–	–	–	+	–
Thielen	1987	+	+	–	+	+	–	+	–
Hillel	1988	+	–	–	–	–	+	+	+
Honda	1988	+	–	–	–	–	–	–	–
Iwata	1988			ADL activities, not specified					
Jerusalem	1988	timed	–	–	–	–	–	–	–
Pinelli	1988	timed	–	–	–	–	–	–	–
Plaitakis	1988	+	–	–	–	–	–	–	–
Total	26	22	13	1	8	8	2	11	3

operationally, and by training raters (Mor et al., 1984). The Glasgow Outcome Scale was devised for head injuries, but may also be suitable for ALS research (Jennet and Bond, 1975). The Rankin scale (Rankin, 1957) is also well known in neurology, and has been used in the European Carotid Trial, the UK-TIA study and recently in the Netherlands TIA-trial, its reliability in stroke patients being good.

QUALITY OF LIFE

The relation between motor capacity, bulbar function, and quality of life is, as yet, unknown. Stensman (1985) has compared the overall quality of life in

Table 18-17. *Activities of Daily Living (ADL)—II*

Author	Year	Feed	Hand function	Write	Hold up head	Fatigability
Norris	1974	+	–	+	+	+
Rivera	1980	–	–	–	–	+
Brooke	1981	–	+	–	–	–
Engel	1983	–	–	–	–	–
Bradley	1984		ADL activities, not specified			
Gracco	1984	–	–	–	–	–
Newrick	1984	+	–	–	–	–
Saida	1984	+	–	+	+	+
Sufit	1984	–	+	–	–	–
Andres	1986	–	–	–	–	–
Brooke	1986	–	–	–	–	–
Caroscio	1986	–	–	–	–	–
Dalakas	1986	+	–	+	+	+
Mitsumoto	1986	–	–	–	–	–
Appel	1987	+	–	–	–	–
Brooks	1987	+	–	+	+	+
Guiloff	1987	+	–	+	+	+
Kuether	1987	+	–	+	+	+
Sinaki	1987	–	–	–	–	–
Thielen	1987	+	–	+	+	+
Hillel	1988	–	–	–	–	–
Honda	1988	–	–	–	–	–
Iwata	1988		ADL activities, not specified			
Jerusalem	1988	–	–	–	–	–
Pinelli	1988	–	–	–	–	–
Plaitakis	1988	–	–	–	–	–
Total	26	9	2	7	7	8

severely mobility-disabled people and in normal controls. The results from both groups did not differ, which may reflect personal adaptation, successful rehabilitation, or compensation by some positive consequences of the disability.

ALS and some of its attempted treatments, such as total lymph node irradiation, may greatly affect the quality of life, yet quality-of-life criteria are seldom used as evaluation endpoints in ALS research; and not at all in any of the 26 assessment protocols considered.

Table 18-18. *Activities of Daily Living (ADL) and Handicap*

Author	Year	ADL Activities	Ability of self-care	Devices needed	Care source
Norris	1974	+	–	–	–
Rivera	1980	+ [a]	–	–	–
Brooke	1981	+	–	+	–
Engel	1983	–	–	–	–
Bradley	1984	+	–	–	–
Gracco	1984	–	–	–	–
Newrick	1984	+	–	–	+
Saida	1984	+	–	–	–
Sufit	1984	+	–	+	–
Andres	1986	+ [a]	–	–	–
Brooke	1986	+ [a]	–	–	–
Caroscio	1986	+ [a]	–	–	–
Dalakas	1986	+	–	–	–
Mitsumoto	1986	+	+	+	–
Appel	1987	+	–	+	–
Brooks	1987	+	–	–	–
Guiloff	1987	+	–	–	–
Kuether	1987	+	–	–	–
Sinaki	1987	+	–	–	–
Thielen	1987	+	–	–	–
Hillel	1988	+	–	+	–
Honda	1988	+ [a]	–	–	–
Iwata	1988	+	+	–	–
Jerusalem	1988	+ [a]	–	–	–
Pinelli	1988	+ [a]	–	–	–
Plaitakis	1988	+ [a]	–	–	–
Total	26	24	2	5	1

[a] Only mobility.

MEASUREMENT OF CENTRAL AND PERIPHERAL MOTOR NEURON INVOLVEMENT

Central Motor Neuron

One major problem in ALS research is how to measure the degree and extent of central motor neuron affection (Table 18-19). It is doubtful whether muscle tone and spasticity are useful predictors, and there is no generally accepted, accurate method of measuring such clinical signs as hyperrflexia, muscle tone, and spasticity. In some indices they are rated according to a subjected grading system, e.g., absent, mild, or severe. The technique of transcranial stimulation (Murray, 1987; Merton and Morton, 1980) offers an opportunity to investigate

Table 18-19. *Neurological Examination*

Author	Year	Reflexes	Muscle atrophy	Fasciculation	Muscle tone	Range of motion
Norris	1974	+	+	+	+	−
Rivera	1980			Not specified		
Brooke	1981	−	−	−	−	+
Engel	1983	+	−	+	+	−
Bradley	1984			Not specified		
Gracco	1984	−	−	−	−	−
Newrick	1984	−	−	−	−	−
Saida	1984	+	+	+	+	−
Sufit	1984	−	−	−	−	+
Andres	1986	−	−	−	−	−
Brooke	1986	−	−	−	−	−
Caroscio	1986	+	−	−	+	−
Dalakas	1986	+	+	+	+	−
Mitsumoto	1986	+	−	−	+	−
Appel	1987	−	−	−	−	−
Brooks	1987	+	+	+	+	−
Guiloff	1987	+	+	+	+	−
Kuether	1987	+	+	+	+	−
Sinaki	1987	−	−	−	−	−
Thielen	1987	+	+	+	+	−
Hillel	1988	−	−	−	−	−
Honda	1988	−	−	−	−	−
Iwata	1988	−	−	−	−	−
Jerusalem	1988	−	−	−	−	−
Pinelli	1988	−	−	−	−	−
Plaitakis	1988	−	−	−	−	−
Total	26	12–10	9–7	10–8	12–10	3–2

excitability and impulse propagation of central neurons. In some ALS patients, Ingram and Swash (1987) have detected a reduction in central conduction time.

In addition, timed motor activities may yield indirect evidence on upper motor neuron function, because spasticity decreases the speed of action and of alternating movements (Sahrmann and Norton, 1977).

Peripheral Motor Neuron Fasciculation

The ratio of rating the severity of fasciculation is doubtful, because its clinical significance for the rate of progression is not clear, due to reflecting both degeneration and regeneration. Fasciculations are a diagnostic sign of peripheral motor neuron involvement and should probably not be included

Table 18-20. *Evaluation of Scientific Quality of Assessment Protocols* —I

Author	Year	Clinical relevance	Correlation with other measurements of outcome	Clinically different phenomena combined	Internal consistency	Reliability	Sensitivity for change (low for ordinal data)
Norris	1974	Good	With force, not survival	+	?	Good	Low
Rivera	1980	?	?	+	?	?	Low
Brooke	1981	Good	?	+	?	Good	Good
Engel	1983	?	?	+	?	?	?
Bradley	1984	?	?	+	?	?	Good
Gracco	1984	?	?	+	?	?	Good
Newrick	1984	Good	Good in CVA	–	?	?	Low
Saida	1984	Good	See Norris	+	?	Good	Low
Sufit	1984	Good	?	+	?	Good	Good
Andres	1986	Good	?	+	+	Good	Good
Brooke	1986	Good	?	+	?	Good	Good
Caroscio	1986	?	?	+	?	?	Good
Dalakas	1986	Good	See Norris	+	?	Good	Low
Mitsumoto	1986	?	?	+	?	?	Good
Appel	1987	Good	With clin. status	+	+	Good	Low
Brooks	1987	Good	See Norris	+	?	Good	Good
Guiloff	1987	Good	See Norris	+	?	Good	Good
Kuther	1987	Good	See Norris	+	?	Good	Good
Sinaki	1987	Good	?	+	?	?	Low
Thielen	1987	Good	See Norris	+	?	Good	Low
Hillel	1988	Good	?	+	?	?	Low
Honda	1988	Good	?	+	?	?	Low
Iwata	1988	Good	?	+	?	?	Low
Jerusalem	1988	Good	?	+	+	Good	Good
Pinelli	1988	?	?	+	?	?	?
Plaitakis	1988	?	?	+	?	?	Low
Satisfactory		18	9	1	3	13	12

in evaluation protocols reflecting progression of the disease. If necessary, fasciculations can be counted by surface recordings (Hjorth et al., 1973).

Table 18-21. *Evaluation of Scientific Quality of Assessment Protocols —II*

Author	Year	Simplicity	Results easily communi-cated	Range of results suf-ficient	Ranks clearly defined & not over-lapping	Used in ther. trials
Norris	1974	+	+	+	–	+
Rivera	1980	–	–	?	?	+
Brooke	1981	–	–	+	+	+
Engel	1983	?	?	?	?	+
Bradley	1984	–	?	?	?	+
Gracco	1984	–	–	?	No ranks	+
Newrick	1984	+	+	+	+	–
Saida	1984	–	–	+	–	+
Sufit	1984	–	–	+	+	+
Andres	1986	–	–	+	No ranks	+
Brooke	1986	–	–	+	No ranks	+
Caroscio	1986	–	–	+	?	+
Dalakas	1986	–	–	+	–	+
Mitsumoto	1986	–	–	+	+	+
Appel	1987	–	–	+	+	+
Brooks	1987	–	–	+	–	+
Guiloff	1987	–	–	+	–	+
Kuether	1987	–	–	+	–	+
Sinaki	1987	+	+	+	–	+
Thielen	1987	–	–	+	–	+
Hillel	1988	+	+	+	+	–
Honda	1988	+	+	+	–	–
Iwata	1988	+	+	+	–	–
Jerusalem	1988	–	–	+	No ranks	+
Pinelli	1988	–	–	–	No ranks	+
Plaitakis	1988	–	–	+	?	+
Total	26	6	6	21	6	22

Muscle Atrophy

Routine clinical methods measuring loss of subcutaneous fat as well as muscle atrophy together do not give information on individual and deep-seated limb muscles, trunk, and bulbar musculature. With the advent of computerized tomography (CT), a new objective method has become available for determining muscular atrophy (Bulcke and Baert, 1982). In ALS, disseminated fatty infiltrates and reduction of muscular cross-sectional areas can be observed (Hawley et al., 1984; Kuether et al., 1987). Planimetric and densitometric calculations allow measurement of deep-seated muscles. Although

Kuether et al., (1987) have demonstrated a good correlation between the CT-parameters and thigh-muscle force of ALS patients, the relation between muscle atrophy and number of motor neurons and strength of most muscle groups is still unknown (Serratrice, 1986). Furthermore, the clinical relevance of muscle atrophy in relation to the progression of the disease and the functional condition of the patient is unclear.

Electrophysiology

Electromyography (EMG) and measurement of nerve conduction velocity are essential diagnostic tools in ALS. In contrast to nerve conduction studies, which serve mainly to exclude other underlying or additional disorders, various EMG techniques, e.g., conventional, single-fiber, and macro-EMG, enable us to measure aspects of deinnervation and reinnervation (Bradley, 1987): amplitude, duration, phases of motor unit potentials, their cross-sectional area, and fiber density.

Unfortunately, quantitation is mainly confined to phenomena secondary to motor neuron loss, i.e., reinnervation by surviving healthy motor neurons As a result, the extent of motoneuron loss must be estimated by crude and indirect means. More direct methods of motor-unit counting employ the principle of calculating the number of stimulated motor units from the compound motor potential (McComas et al., 1974; McComas, 1977; Ballentyne and Hansen, 1974). Only small distal muscles can be investigated, but Strong et al. (1988) have now attempted to study proximal muscles.

All these electrophysiological methods have the disadvantages of being confined to a few selected muscles and being time consuming as well as inconvenient to the patient. In addition, the relation between EMG and motor function, functional capacity, and survival is still unknown. As with all our present in-vivo methods, EMG watches the smoke rather than the fire. Nevertheless, electrophysiology provides the only access to the processes of motor neuron loss and muscle-fiber reinnervation (see Chapter 17). For this reason, protocols on pathogenesis will require more emphasis on EMG than has been customary, although, in therapeutic trials, electrophysiological findings are of secondary value because the correlation with disease progression is unknown.

DISCUSSION

Review of the literature has disclosed a broad consensus that we should at least rate strength, bulbar function, and pulmonary capacity, but how to do so is a matter of controversy. Two reliable methods of force measurement are strain-gauge myometry, e.g., The Tufts Quantitative Neuromuscular Examination (Andres et al., 1986) and hand-held myometry (Wiles, 1983; van der Ploeg and Oosterhuis, 1984). To date, the only validated and reliable index of bulbar function is the Frenchay Dysarthria Assessment (Enderby, 1983). Because pulmonologists have created extensive databanks on normal respiratory function, it is easy to select those tests that do not require intact functioning of the orofacial musculature (Norris and Fallat, 1988; Kuether, 1987).

ADL and handicap scales will assist in better revealing our patients' needs and will allow the procurement of the necessary aids, without the usual delay currently seen.

Faced with the necessity of starting a controlled, prospective, therapeutic trial in the autumn of 1988, we (Louwerse and De Jong) chose to employ hand-held myometry, the Frenchay Dysarthria Index, portable spirometry, the Rankin ADL Scale, and the Barthel Handicap Index (Tables 18-20 and 18-21).

A common international ALS rating system would enable researchers to determine the efficacy of symptomatic treatment, yield knowledge of its natural history and the effect of placebo treatment, and will minimize the necessity of double-blind placebo-controlled trials. The time to act is now.

Acknowledgment: E. S. Louwerse acknowledges partial support by the Netherlands ALS Society. We are grateful for the advice, help, and hospitality received in Bonn from Prof. F. Jerusalem and Ms. J. Fresmann, in Bristol from Dr. R. Langton Hewer and Ms. P. Enderby. We thank Prof. Th. Munsat and Ms. P. Andrews for assistance and information on the Tufts Quantitative Neuromuscular Assessment, Drs. F. H. Norris and E. Denys for discussion and advice, and Prof. S. Conradi for his kind permission to print Fig. 18-1.

REFERENCES

Andres PL, Hedlund W, Finison L, Conlon T, Felmus M, Munsat TL. Quantitative motor assessment in amyotrophic lateral sclerosis. *Neurology* 1986;36:937–41.

Andres PL, Thibodeau LM, Finison LJ, Munsat TL. Quantitative assessment of neuromuscular deficit in ALS. *Neurol Clin* 1987;5:125–41.

Andrews K, Stewart J. Stroke recovery: he can but does he? *Rheumatol Rehab* 1979;18:43–8.

Appel V, Stewart SS, Smith G, Appel SH. A rating scale for amyotrophic lateral sclerosis: description and preliminary experience. *Ann Neurol* 1987;22:328–33.

Appel SH, Stewart SS, Appel V, Harati Y, Mietlowski W, Weiss W, Belundiuk GW. A double-blind study of the effectiveness of cyclosporine in amyotrophic lateral sclerosis. *Arch Neurol* 1988;45:381–6.

Ballentyne JP, Hansen S. A new method for the estimation of the number of motor units in a muscle. *J Neurol Neurosurg Psychiatry* 1974;37:907–15.

Barlow SM, Abbs JH. Orafacial fine motor control impairment in congenital spastics: evidence against muscle spindle related performance deficits. *Neurology* 1984;34:145–50.

Beasly WC. Quantitative muscle testing: principles and application to research and clinical services. *Arch Phys Med Rehabil* 1961;42:398–425.

Boer A de, Boukes RJ, Sterk JC. Reliability of dynametry in patients with a neuromuscular disorder. *Eng Med* 1982;11:169–74.

Bradley WG, Hedlund W, Cooper C, et al. A double-blind controlled trial of bovine brain gangliosides in amyotrophic lateral sclerosis. *Neurology* 1984;34:1079–82.
Bradley WG. Recent views on amyotrophic lateral sclerosis with emphasis on electrophysiological studies. *Muscle Nerve* 1987;10:490–502.
Brooke MH, Griggs RC, Mendell JR, Fenichel GM, Shumate JB, Pellegrino RJ. Clinical trial in Duchenne dystrophy. I. The design of the protocol. *Muscle Nerve* 1981;4:186–97.
Brooke MH, Florence JM, Heller SL, Kaiser KK, Phillips D, Gruber A, Babcock D, Miller JP. Controlled trial of thyrotropin releasing hormone in amyotrophic lateral sclerosis. *Neurology* 1986;36:146–51.
Brooks BR, Sufit RL, Montgomery GK, Beaulieu DA, Erickson LM. Intraveneous thyrotropin-releasing hormone in patients with amyotrophic lateral sclerosis. *Neurol Clin* 1987;5,1:143–56.
Bulcke JAL, Baert AL. *Clinical and radiological aspects of myopathies.* Berlin, Heidelberg, New York: Springer Verlag, 1982.
Caroscio JT, Cohen JA, Zawodniak J, et al. A double-blind, placebo-controlled trial of TRH in amyotrophic lateral sclerosis. *Neurology* 1986;36:141–5.
Cohen JA, Gundesblatt M, Miller A, et al. Predictive value of pulmonary function testing in ALS. *Neurology* 1985;35:72.
Dalakas MC, Aksamit AJ, Madden DL, Sever JL. Administration of recombinant human leucocyte alpha2-interferon in patients with amyotrophic lateral sclerosis. *Arch Neurol* 1986;43:933–5.
Dalakas MC, Elder G, Hallett M, et al. A long-term folloe-up study of patients with postpoliomyelitis neuromuscular symptoms. *N Engl J Med* 1986;31:959–93.
Donaldson SW, Wagner CC, Gresham GE. A unified ADL evaluation form. *Arch Phys Med Rehabli* 1973;54:175–9.
Dubowitz V, Heckmatt JZ, Hyde SA, Gabain A. Therapeutic trial of isaxonine in Duchenne muscular dystrophy. *Muscle Nerve* 1986;9:270.
Enderby PM. *Frenchay dysarthria assessment.* San Diego: College-Hill Press, 1983.
Engel WK, Siddique T, Nicoloff JT. Effect on weakness and spasticity in amyotrophic lateral sclerosis of thyrotropin-releasing hormone. *Lancet* 1983;1:73–5.
Fallat RJ, Jewitt, Bass M, Kamm B, Norris FH. Spirometry in amyotrophic lateral sclerosis. *Arch Neurol* 1979;36:74–80.
Feinstein AR. *Clinimetrics.* New Haven and London: Yale University Press, 1987:3.
Gracco VL, Caliguiri M, Abbs JH, Sufit L, Brooks BR. Placebo controlled computerized dynametric measurements of bulbar and somatic muscle strength increase in patients with amyotrophic lateral sclerosis following intravenous infusion of 10 mg/kg thyrotropin-releasing hormone. *Ann Neurol* 1984;16:110.
Gresham GE, Phillips TF, Labi MLC. ADL status in stroke: relative merits of three standard indexes. *Arch Phys Med Rehabil* 1980;61:355–8.
Griggs RC, Donahue KM, Utell MJ, et al. Evaluation of pulmonary function in neuromuscular disease. *Arch Neurol* 1981;38:9–12.
Guiloff RJ, Eckland DJA. Observations in the clinical assessment of patients with motor neuron disease. *Neurol Clin* 1987;5:171–92.
Hawley RJ, Schellinger D, O'Doherty DS. Computed tomographic patterns of muscles in neuromuscular diseases. *Arch Neurol* 1984;41:383–7.

Hillel AD, Miller RM, McDonald E, Konikow N, Norris FH. ALS severity scale. In: Tsubaki T, Yase Y, eds. *Amyotrophic lateral sclerosis. Recent advances in research and treatment.* Amsterdam: Excerpta Medica, 1988:247–52.

Hjorth RJ, Walsh JC, Willison RG. The distribution and frequency of spontaneous fasciculations in motor neuron disease. *J Neurol Sci* 1973;18:469–74.

Honda M. Clinical strategies in dealing with ALS. In: Tsubaki T, Yase Y, eds. *Amyotrophic lateral sclerosis. Recent advances in research and treatment.* Amsterdam: Excerpta Medica, 1988:207–9.

Ingram DA, Swash M. Central motor conduction is abnormal in motor neuron disease. *J Neurol Neurosurg Psychiatry* 1987;50:159–66.

Iwata M. Clinical management of ALS according to the severity stage. In: Tsubaki T, Yase Y, eds. *Amyotrophic lateral sclerosis. Recent advances in research and treatment.* Amsterdam: Excerpta Medica, 1988:223–9.

Jennett B, Bond M. Assessment of outcome after severe brain damage; a practical scale. *Lancet* 1975;1:480–4.

Jerusalem F, Fresmann J, Sayn H, Schulz G. A double-blind, placebo controlled trial of bestatin in amyotrophic lateral sclerosis (ALS). In: Tsubaki T, Yase Y, eds. *Amyotrophic lateral sclerosis. Recent advances in research and treatment. Amsterdam: Excerpta Medica, 1988:333–8.*

Karnofsky DA, Burchenal JH. Clinical evaluation of chemotherapeutic agents in cancer. In: MacLeod CM, ed. *Evaluation of chemotherapeutic agents.* New York: Columbia University Press, 1949.

Katz S, Ford AB, Moskowitz RW, Jackson BA, Jaffe MW. Studies of illness in the aged. The index of ADL: a standardized measure of biological and psychosocial function. *J Am Med Assoc* 1963;185:914–9.

Kuether G, Rodiek SO, Struppler A. CT-scanning of skeletal muscles in amyotrophic lateral sclerosis. In: Cosi V, Kato AC, Parlette W, Pinelli P, Poloni M, eds. *Amyotrophic lateral sclerosis. Therapeutic, psychological and research aspects. Advances in experimental medicine and biology*, vol 209. New York: Plenum Press, 1987:143–8.

Kuether G, Struppler A. Therapeutic trial with *N*-acetylcystein in amyotrophic lateral sclerosis. In: Cosi V, Kato AC, Parlette W, Pinelli P, Poloni M, eds. *Amyotrophic lateral sclerosis. Therapeutic, psychological and research aspects. Advances in experimental medicine and biology*, vol 209. New York: Plenum Press, 1987:281–4.

Kuether G, Struppler A, Lipinski HG. Therapeutic trials in ALS — the design of a protocol. In Cosi V, Kato AC, Parlette W, Pinelli P, Poloni M, eds. *Amyotrophic lateral sclerosis. Therapeutic, psychological and research aspects. Advances in experimental medicine and biology*, vol 209. New York: Plenum Press, 1987:265–76.

Mahoney FI, Barthel DW. Functional evaluation: the Barthel index. *Maryland State Med J* 1965;14:61–5

McComas AJ. *Neuromuscular function and disorders*, London: Butterworths, 1977.

McComas AJ, Fawcett PPW, Cambell MJ, Sica REP. Electrophysiological estimation of the number of motor units within hand muscle. *J Neurol Neurosurg Psychiatry* 1974;34:121–31.

Medical Research Council. Aids to the investigation of the peripheral nerve injuries. *War Memorandum*, 2nd ed. (revised). London: HSMO, 1943:11–46.

Merton PA, Morton HB. Stimulation of the cerebral cortex in the intact human subject. *Nature* 1980;285:227.

Mitsumoto H, Salgado ED, Negroski D, et al. Amyotrophic lateral sclerosis: effect of acute intravenous and chronic subcutaneous administration of thyrotropin-releasing hormone in controlled trials. *Neurology* 1986;36:152–9.

Mor V, Laliberte L, Morris JN. The Karnofsky performance status scale: an examination of its reliability and validity in research setting. *Cancer* 1984;53:2002–7.

Murray NMF. Clinical uses of electrical and magnetic stimulation *EEG J* 1987:70s.

Newrick PG, Langton Hewer R. Motor neurone disease: can we do better? A study of 42 patients. *Br Med J* 1984;289:539–42.

Norris FH, Calanchini PR, Fallat RJ, Panacharis S, Jewett B. The administration of guanidine in amyotrophic lateral sclerosis. *Neurology* 1974;24:721–8.

Norris FH, Denys EH, Fallat RJ. Trial of octacosanol in amyotrophic lateral sclerosis. *Neurology* 1986;36:1263–4.

Norris FH, Fallat RJ. Staging respiratory failure in ALS. In: Tsubaki T, Yase Y, eds. *Amyotrophic lateral sclerosis. Recent advances in research and treatment.* Amsterdam: Excerpta Medica, 1988: 217–22.

Pinelli P. The effect of repeated doses of TRH on sick motor units of ALS patients. In: Tsubaki T, Yase Y, eds. *Amyotrophic lateral sclerosis. Recent advances in research and treatment.* Amsterdam: Excerpta Medica, 1988:307–12.

Plaitakis A, Smith J, Mandeli J, Yahr MD. Pilot trial of branched-chain aminoacids in amyotrophic lateral sclerosis. *Lancet* 1988;1:1015–8.

Ploeg RJO van der, Oosterhuis HJGH, Reuvekamp J. Measuring muscle strength. *J Neurol* 1984;231:200–3.

Rankin J. Cerebral vascular accidents in patients over the age of 60. 2. Prognosis. *Scott Med J* 1957;2:200–15.

Riviera VM, Grabois M, Deaton W, Breitbach W, Hines M. Modified snake venom in ALS. Lack of clinical effectiveness. *Arch Neurol* 1980;37:201–3.

Sahrmann SA, Norton BJ. The relationship of voluntary movement of spasticity in the upper motor neuron syndrome. *Ann Neurol* 1977;2:460–5.

Saida T, Imoto K, Saida K, Iwamura K, Nishitani H. Trial of thyrotropin-releasing hormone treatment of patients with amyotrophic lateral sclerosis. *Ann Neurol* 1984;16:109.

Sanguq M, Paulson D, Sufit RL, et al. inefficient increased oxygen consumption during submaximal exercise in amyotrophic lateral sclerosis. *Ann Neurol* 1984;16:110.

Sanjak M, Paulson D, Sufit R, Reddan W, Beaulieu D, Erickson L, Shug A, Brooks BR. Physiologic and metabolic reponse to progressive and prolonged exercise in amyotrophic lateral sclerosis. *Neurology* 1987;37:1217–20.

Schag CC, Heinrich RL, Ganz PA. Karnofsky performance status revisited: reliability, validity and guidelines. *J Clin Oncol* 1984;2:187–93.

Serratrice G. Computed tomography of muscles in neuromuscular disease. In: Dimitrijevic MR, Kakulas BA, Vrbova G, eds. *Recent achievements in restorative neurology. 2. Progressive neuromuscular diseases.* London: Karger, 1986: 156–69.

Sinaki M, Litchy JW, Mulder DW. Motor neuron disease. In: Johnson RT, ed. *Current therapy in neurologic disease 2.* Oxford: Blackwell Scientific, 1987:255–8.

Amyotrophic Lateral Sclerosis,
edited by F. Clifford Rose.
Demos Publications, New York © 1990.

19

Special Problems of Physiotherapy Trials in Motor Neuron Disease

A. S. Brooke and T. J. Steiner

Academic Unit of Neuroscience, Charing Cross and Westminster Medical School, London, England

Trials to evaluate physiotherapy in motor neuron disease (MND) face many exceptional obstacles, and controlled experiments are unusually difficult. Posed by the illness itself is its variability (with three clinical subtypes) in terms of areas of the body affected and degree of weakness, the type of weakness, and the rate of progression. Accurate, objective testing is problematic in all neuromuscular disease and MND brings additional problems of cramps, painful joints, and excess fatigue to a variable baseline. A representative patient group is difficult to find in one geographically limited center, and diagnostic biases threaten when many patients are either self-referring or tertiary referrals from other centers.

Most patients will have developed individual strategies for coping that hinder standardization of therapy, much of which, good and bad, depends on the qualities of their caregivers. The same strategies may themselves be hindered by admission to the hospital, with the deleterious effects of this offsetting the presumed advantage brought by the therapeutic intervention. The usual need to follow up patients necessitates home visits so that patients can be assessed where they normally function, and without the need for repeated travel to the hospital, perhaps over long distances. Control groups require patients to receive, and perhaps be admitted for, bogus therapy, presenting ethical problems in the face of a progressive fatal disease.

Physiotherapy itself is difficult to standardize, and has to be tailored to individual needs. It is therefore an intervention with many subjective effects that are difficult to monitor and others attributable to placebo effect and to the interest taken. Compliance with therapy is usually good in the absence of side effects but long term programs require motivation of patient and family in the face of relentless deterioration. Availability of physiotherapy in the community cannot be guaranteed in quantity or quality. Because of this, and the expense of physiotherapy, cost/benefit judgments must be among a trial's objectives so that effective therapy can be allocated appropriate priority (neither too much nor too little) in the competition for limited resources.

OVERVIEW

Physiotherapy is a discipline in which objective research is difficult because of the nature of the intervention. The double-blind conditions of drug trials cannot be reproduced for a therapy that depends on patient–therapist interaction, nor can physiotherapy be dispensed in fixed doses within a standard regimen. It is nonetheless extremely important that studies are done, to be sure of what is optimal patient care, not least because physiotherapy is an expensive and scarce resource. Basmajian (1) said, "Almost all therapeutic procedures in rehabilitation departments must be regarded with suspicion; it is sound science to start on the premise that they may be either useless or harmful. The science behind them is not as strong as the faith."

In MND this problem is compounded by the variable symptoms and signs that present or develop, the relentless but inconsistent progression, and the range of possible physiotherapeutic interventions. There is considerable controversy over the value of exercise in MND. Claims include "astonishing recoveries" from daily exercise alone (2). Others warn that weakness may become apparent for the first time with exercise and continue afterwards (3). Therapeutic objectives must depend on the patient and, in some, energy should rather be preserved for essential activities of daily living. When it is not possible to restore full function, realistic aims are to maximize residual function and improve physical comfort.

GENERAL ISSUES

"Special problems" of physiotherapy trials in MND therefore stem from the specific issues — related to the disease, the patients, and the therapy, but general issues of clinical trials, those of science, ethics, and judgments of cost/benefit also apply. The extent to which these, too, can produce special problems in the physiotherapy of MND is a matter for discussion here.

Scientific problems arise from the usual need for good experimental design and objective assessments, but obtain special significance in this area because both are unusually difficult to achieve. Standardization of therapy is a contradiction of the philosophy behind all forms of remedial therapy. If therapy is not standardized, can the assessments be? If these are not, what manner of comparative trial is possible? The tendency for investigators in this field to resort to limited-value single-case studies is easily understood.

Ethical issues abound in the study of numbers of terminally ill patients, many of whom in desperation will try anything. This frees potential investigators of those constraints normally imposed by patients' informed consent (i.e., what patients will not, in more normal circumstances, willingly allow to be done to them). It also creates tensions over allocation of patients to untreated comparative groups. These issues are not "special" to physiotherapy trials because they apply to all trials in MND, and they do not obtain particular significance from the fact that physiotherapy may be ineffective or harmful (which is just as true of other trial therapies). The special ethical problem is that resources may not be available for the treatment to continue even if found successful, because physiotherapy is, unfortunately, expensive.

This leads to cost/benefit judgments, and the almost unanswerable question of what cost society should bear to postpone death of an individual, or to improve quality of life until a foreseeable death, assuming either of those benefits is attainable. What cost should society bear for merely a reasonable prospect of such benefits? Domiciliary physiotherapy is very expensive but relatively few physiotherapists might meet the needs of all MND patients because the disease is rare. Does that increase the obligation on society (lower cost), or make it lower priority (benefit to fewer)? If these questions are generated because of a trial outcome, that trial has a duty also to provide the data that enable correct answers to be given. Otherwise it creates a new ethical problem.

The ethics in this situation are mixed with the ethics of limited health care resources, a reality faced to a greater or lesser extent by all societies. Cost containment in the treatment of a disease is an ethical requirement in itself because others, with other illnesses, supposedly will inherit the benefit of freed resources. The "value" of a treatment such as physiotherapy can therefore be measured in these terms: Does it reduce other costs of treating MND? If it helps maintain mobility and independence it may have just this effect, reducing the need for other domiciliary services or residential care. Even in the terminal stages, optimal management of end-stage chest infection at home should prevent costly (and traumatic) hospital admissions. There is an opportunity cost, i.e., the fact that therapists engaged in treating MND patients cannot then be treating others, which is important when therapists themselves are in short supply. More important is the recognizable truth that extending the life of an MND patient generally increases treatment costs.

There are also costs to be borne by the patient, or by other members of the family rather than society at large, and these extend the cost/benefit issue beyond ethics. If physiotherapy is of potential benefit, it becomes a competitor against the purchase of aids, and other sources of increased comfort or improved function. Not enough has been done to assess the value of physiotherapy generally, and it is often difficult to suggest appropriate measures of gain. In the case of young patients with orthopedic conditions, for example, return to work is a criterion that measures the achievement in terms of economic relevance to both patient and society. MND can sometimes give rise to a similar situation, especially when falls are caused and lead to secondary injury. Specific physiotherapy in these cases, and provision of appropriate mobility aids in others, may keep a patient at work, but both are special cases. For elderly patients, or those whose illness has progressed beyond the ability to work, achievement is not in these terms. In the absence of economic markers, acknowledging consumer sovereignty is one approach to assessing the value of an intervention; i.e., allowing the receiver of the service to be the best judge of its value. It may be very nonspecific: although in many cases patients may derive (and assess) benefit from the specialist skills of the physiotherapist, what is sometimes valued is simply the chance to discuss problems with someone knowledgeable about the disease.

The role of the physiotherapist in MND is often advisory and preventative, averting possible complications. These gains may not be apparent to the patient. In other ways, too, as stated by Frazer (4), "It is often the relative that experiences greatest benefit from a visit by the domiciliary physiotherapist." Thus, the patient is not the sole receiver of the service that physiotherapy, especially domiciliary physiotherapy, provides, just as the patient is not the sole bearer, within the family, of the cost. If a group study of regular physiotherapy finds, say, marked benefit in 50% of patients, moderate benefit in 25%, and none in 25%, how does the spouse of an affected patient estimate the probability of benefit to one individual and decide whether to continue the therapy at their own cost and at the price of taking their children out of private school (for example)? The reason why this problem is especially relevant to physiotherapy trials in MND is that the particular natures of disease and therapy seem to allow matching of one to the other. This, therefore, adds to the basic objective of these trials: to learn not only whether patients as a group can expect to gain from physiotherapy as opposed to no physiotherapy, or from intensive physiotherapy against routine, but also which patients have the greatest expectation of benefit and, for costing purposes, from what sort of physiotherapy, and how much of it gives the best cost/benefit ratio.

SPECIFIC ISSUES

The Disease

Variability

The variable nature of MND is well known. It presents in many ways, each differing in symptoms and signs. According to Rose (5), one-third of patients have bulbar symptoms at onset (progressive bulbar palsy; PBP) but in the majority distal weakness, of either upper or lower limbs, comes first. Occasionally several areas of the body appear to develop weakness simultaneously, and respiratory problems can initiate medical referral (6). Fifteen percent of patients (5) develop purely lower-motor-neuron weakness (PMA), whereas others develop a mixed pattern of upper and lower-motor-neuron involvement (amyotrophic lateral sclerosis; ALS). Prognosis is more than correspondingly variable because progression, although always inexorable with a mean survival time dependent on disease type, can in all cases be fast or slow. PBP patients have an average survival time of 2 years, and PMA and ALS patients have 6 and 4 years survival, respectively (5).

Wide variations in the rate and pattern of disease progression that cannot be predicted create enormous difficulties for studies of effects of intervention. For physiotherapy trials, major problems are also introduced by the need always to have the therapy appropriately adapted to the state of the patient. Sometimes the therapy itself must be constantly changing. Using quantitative and sensitive techniques of measuring neuromuscular function in 50 patients with both upper and lower-motor-neuron involvement, Munsat et al. (7) found deterioration rates indicative of motor neuron loss to be remarkably linear. Andres et al. (8), using the Tufts Quantitative Neuromuscular Examination, found an average deterioration of 4.5% per month. The rate of deterioration in these terms may be linear, but at critical times small decrements in muscle power cause major functional losses, and decline with heterogeneous patterns of disease.

Assessment of Outcome

This implies measurement of the patient before and after intervention and perhaps during it as well. Single-case studies are an approach that sidesteps the difficulties of measuring in terms applicable to a group of patients for between-group comparisons. These are a special type of trial, particularly suited to remedial therapy. In many ways they have been developed as an alternative method to avoid the problems described here, so they shall not be further discussed.

The disease affects the integrity of nerve cells but manifests principally as loss of muscle power, and patients complain of loss of a range of functional abilities. Assessment of outcome therefore implies measurement of these. Death of a patient is an outcome too, measurable in absolute terms or in terms of time until it happens. These ultimate measures have some application in the study of physiotherapy, but principally to special procedures such as chest drainage.

Accurate and objective assessment of the neuromuscular system is so difficult, especially the monitoring of muscle strength and tone, that no one has described a definitive way of doing it. Muscle power can be assessed using the Medical Research Council (9) grading system, scoring 0–5, but its use is limited by insensitivity, subjectivity, and wide variations between grades. Dynamometry with, for example, the Penny and Giles electromyometer (10), produces accurate and reproducible results with correct use. Strain gauges can give objective measurements of isometric (static) muscle force (7), but isometric contractions produce muscle cramps in many MND patients; results are invalidated when this happens. Isokinetic equipment (LIDO or Cybex) tests human muscle performance isokinetically throughout the range of movement, measuring strongest and weakest parts of the range at preset speeds. Isokinetic work is defined as dynamic muscle activity performed at constant angular velocity (11). These systems are accurate and objective, but are unsuitable for testing severe weakness because of their inertia, and positioning of heavily disabled patients on the apparatus is difficult. Other equipment measures unrestrained human movement rather than muscle force (e.g., polarized light goniometry, CODA-3). Goniometry during movement, in expert hands, undoubtedly aids the recognition of certain problems despite a lack of published reports of its use. CODA-3, which is able to analyze movement with a high degree of precision in three dimensions, has not yet been found useful in MND, mainly because suitable paradigms have still to be developed for its use. All of these systems are costly and unsuitable for home assessment.

To these difficulties MND adds its own. Muscle testing in MND patients is hampered by painful joints and muscle contractures, spasticity and cramps, dyspnea, fatigue, poor communication, and emotional lability. Muscle power in MND is subject to fluctuations during the day and from day to day. A poor night's rest, a hot bath, or even constipation, all affect performance.

MND affects muscle tone as much as power. When the result is spasticity, physiotherapy is expected to be able to help. Testing spasticity as resistance to passive movement in the limbs is always clinically difficult, largely unhelped by technology, and in any case not necessarily relevant to its effect on function. Body position and emotional state are two of the many factors that alter muscle tone even with standardization of medication taken to reduce spasticity.

Contractures can be measured, and their effects on gait can be monitored. Gait is fortunately objectively quantifiable in many ways, although good measures of quality of gait remain elusive. This, at least, is a function the measure of which is relevant to the illness, and to physiotherapy as a treatment of the illness, although not to all patients. Gait is soon lost in many patients but is unimpaired in a few, and in all cases other functional losses occur.

Scores of "overall" function are available (e.g., 8,12,13). They are nonlinear and difficult to repeat accurately at home, where function most needs to be measured. Many factors affecting functional assessment are subjective, and some of these are important goals in themselves for the physiotherapist, although they are virtually impossible to quantify. The patient may feel more comfortable at night after prescribed exercise, or may experience less pain in the shoulder. Sensory pathways remain intact in MND and musculoskeletal aches and pains are common (14,15) as secondary effects of immobility. Some patients after physiotherapy report feeling "less stiff" in the mornings.

Especially in terminal disease for which little other help is offered, patients are responsive to the placebo effect of individual care and attention. Placebo may give rise to objective improvements in muscle power and performance through increased voluntary effort, and the primary effects of physiotherapy can then be quite difficult to separate.

Practicalities of Treatment and Follow-up

The central feature of MND is progressively increasing disability, eventually becoming severe in all cases. Disabled patients often cannot endure traveling long distances for assessment and therapy, or do so at considerable cost to them. Rarely can they do so repeatedly. This may cause hospital admission for these purposes, but a stay of any length may be detrimental in its own way. The patient's routine is upset. Disturbances at night, altered diet, and enforced inactivity affect health and mobility. Single wards may help if available, but aids to improve mobility or electric beds and elevating chairs, however thoughtfully provided, never replicate home. A clutter of strategically placed pieces of furniture may be the key to a patient's movement about the house. Inhibited for too long by its not being there, the patient may never recover. Conversely, the benefits from the particular care and attention available in the hospital, and rest from the fraught situations that can occur at home, may foster improvements independent of the therapy under evaluation.

For the serial assessments that this progressive disease may call for, patients whose disability is increasing are unlikely to remain willing or able to return continually to the hospital, even if they were initially. Home visits are an answer to this problem (A. S. Brooke and T. J. Steiner, unpublished observations). They are costly, and testing does not take place under standardized conditions, but patients have use of those aids that actually determine their performance at home. Equally relevant to assessment are thick pile carpets that impede mobility at home, and beds and chairs of the wrong height for easy transfers. Ignoring these factors in the name of standardized assessments is nonsense. Equally important to an assessment may be direct observation of the provision of services, and of interfamily relationships.

The Patients

Selection Bias

Because MND is a rare condition, trials may need to recruit from a large geographical area. The resulting requirement to travel considerable distances may deter the attendance especially of those with advanced disease. In the United Kingdom, no means of access exists to a random representative sample of those with MND. To any major center, referral is mostly tertiary, from other neurological centers, or self-generated through agencies such as the Motor Neurone Disease Association. Most patients with an established diagnosis will be listed in hospital units somewhere, although by no means necessarily neurological, and with their general practitioners, but there are many for whom the diagnosis has not been made, is incorrect or not imparted, and many others who have not yet sought medical help. Nobody knows how these factors bias entry to trials, or even whether it matters. Still other patients do not wish to take part in research, whereas the opposite extreme — patients desperate to try anything, consenting to everything, however offered, and if possible all at once — is commonly encountered. As far as trials of physiotherapy are concerned, patients may have views of their own on its likely benefit (more than would be the case with a drug treatment), and those offering themselves will be those with expectation of benefit (rightly or wrongly).

Elderly patients and those with young dependents will be less likely to take part in demanding studies, which those of physiotherapy may be. Patient associations such as the Motor Neurone Disease Association are unrepresentative in geographical distribution and social class. A sample will poorly represent those still working and therefore unwilling to take time off work repeatedly. This may also reflect social class, but may exclude those most highly motivated. Conversely, patients in whom the disease provokes depression, perhaps highly represented in a particular subgroup, will not be motivated to take part.

Individual Problems and Strategies

Giant hurdles to scientific study are created by the variable nature of the disease, but patients' differing adaptations to their illness add more. Disabling neurological diseases create specific difficulties in the handling and positioning of patients, who develop individual strategies, for example, for transfers, with their caregivers. Provision of an aid or demonstration of a technique expected to be helpful can unexpectedly impede such a strategy, and produce functional decline if not rejected. Patients' individualities can in this way be said to interfere with treatment. They can also interfere with assessment. Thus, physical testing may be impaired by patients' inability to lie supine due to dyspnea or back pain, or on their side because of shoulder pain. This may be compounded by a range of other problems, such as arthritic joints or cardiovascular or pulmonary afflictions, that are not part of MND but more age related.

The caregiver, too, is part of this "problem." Independently of the character of the disease, patients are generally advantaged, often greatly, if living with a close relative, especially a spouse and usually more when the spouse is the wife. This is not always the case, and sometimes a more distant relative or friend, perhaps living elsewhere, provides redress. However, an overattentive or too protective caregiver inhibits strategy-forming and independence, and can in the long term cause more harm than good. When physical function is the target of therapy, this factor can be crucially significant.

Controls

The need for a controlled experiment is unarguable. In the context of clinical trials, this usually means recruiting and following an untreated group of similar patients. Identifying such a group may not be easy because of the issues discussed immediately above. Variability is a problem for all trials, but individual coping strategies fundamentally influence functional capacity and, therefore, the objective of physiotherapy. A "matched" group may have no real meaning in this context.

There are other very serious problems. It is ethically difficult to justify admitting patients to the hospital for extended periods, if that is what the trial demands, without offering any therapy. This is particularly so when, for some patients, admission is itself deleterious (see Practicalities of Treatment and Follow-up). Even when no harm comes of it, for patients with a life expectancy of a few months, two weeks spent in the hospital can be a major sacrifice. Few patients will volunteer for placebo therapy. A comparison of two treatments, both on trial, is possible — physiotherapy perhaps with thyrotrophin-releasing hormone medication—but without placebo control may still be difficult to analyze. Matching for age, sex, disease subtype, stage of disease and rate of progression, areas affected, functional consequences, psychological adjustment and response and coping abilities, impossible in a small and heterogeneous population, makes heavy demands of randomization. Unfortunately, with patients wanting to choose their therapy, or to have the "benefit" of both, randomization too, may be impossible. A control group can be sought in another center that is admitting patients for a similar period for other reasons, not including remedial therapy, to monitor both positive and negative effects of the inpatient stay. This is feasible if testing can be standardized and interventions at the second center have neither beneficial nor deleterious consequences in the period of observation (e.g., are strictly limited to assessment). Unfortunately, a group of patients recruited in this way is an unlikely match for those referred for treatment.

During long-term follow-up, many more uncontrollable factors are introduced. Not only is local availability of physiotherapy unpredictable, varying with time and place, but so is the provision of aids and equipment and the whole range of community services support. The good and bad influences of the caregiver (see Individual Problems and Strategies), whose well-balanced help with prescribed exercise and passive movements especially may be necessary, grow over time. All of these, therefore, at least potentially, are major variables between patients. Add them to the differing courses of the illness, making demands on these services at different times and with different urgency, and to the widely ranging level of family support and problems with the individual patient's general health, and the impediments to usual standards of control become insuperable. According to Munsat et al. (7), longevity is as dependent on "external" health factors such as emphysema, smoking history, general medical care, and respiratory support as on actual motor neuron loss. It is left only to argue that, against the background of chronic, progressive, incurable disease, patients can act as their own controls, and to question whether, in such a context, placebo effect has any lasting power.

The Therapy

Variability: Quantity and Quality

One major difficulty with physiotherapy — its availability or not in the community — is identified above. It is not just a question of local case loads, resources, and budgets at a time of limitation: physiotherapy in particular is dependent on personal skill. Buying it privately is an option for some if domiciliary physiotherapy is not otherwise made available, but even this may be less beneficial, at obviously higher cost, than relying on the services of a caring and expertly instructed spouse if the therapist has general but no special training. Therapists' skill is as intrusive a factor in physiotherapy given in the hospital, but presumably no more than is the surgeon's skill in operative treatments. Like surgical trials, remedial therapy trials adapt themselves readily only to showing what *can* be achieved with best effort in a center having a particular interest. Their outcome should be regarded, and should determine practice elsewhere, in that light. This can be important for cost/benefit analysis (see above).

As important in the conduct of trials is that physiotherapy cannot be dispensed in fixed doses. Equally, physiotherapy is difficult to standardize, both as a short course and, especially, in a long-term program. Treatment always involves patient-therapist interaction, which is not easily quantified and is also variable qualitatively. Physiotherapy involves close physical contact, its core being the therapist's hands (16).

Specifically relevant to MND, each patient has a unique package of therapeutic requirements, both in degree and distribution. Therapy programs and aids provided with them must be tailored to the individual. Much depends on the objectives of the therapy, which differ not only between patients but also within-patient over time. Patients with contractures, spasticity, and poor balance and those with flaccid weakness require quite different management, and severity of these problems and their rate of progression also affect the type of intervention. Different treatment modalities can be employed for the same problem — e.g., shoulder stiffness may benefit from exercise, manipulation, electrotherapy, hydrotherapy, or the use of reflex-inhibiting postures (17) when spasticity is present. Which is most appropriate can be a matter of opinion, and there can be changes in treatment during a long-term course as other therapists with different approaches become involved.

So wide-ranging may the appropriate form of treatment be that it becomes obvious that "physiotherapy" is as loose a term as "medical therapy." Trials involving the latter usually center on a specific dose of a particular drug. Discussion of physiotherapy is thus set at an altogether different level, as is trial design accordingly.

Compliance

Cooperation with assessment and physiotherapy programs is usually not a problem initially, with most MND patients eager to help themselves and participate fully. Compliance with a particular regimen of treatment can be affected by its side-effects. With physiotherapy these are increased fatigue, muscle cramps, and fasciculations. During therapy these effects should be carefully monitored, and the program modified accordingly. Therapy in the hospital is closely supervised but, if the patients are to continue at home, maintained motivation is needed in the face of relentless deterioration. Some exercises require assistance from the caregiver when their time, energy, and patience are already stretched. Supervision by physiotherapy staff in the community is subject to the limitations discussed above, determined by their caseload, their own motivation, and their often slight experience of the disease.

The start of a treatment program for an incurable disease risks hopes being inappropriately raised with the proposition that therapy can help. Unrealistically high expectations can lead later to anger, frustration, and disillusion, as seen in terminal cancer patients (18). This promotes the growth of noncompliance and, with time, artificially poor retest results.

The opposite side of the coin is sometimes seen: patients who argue that "more of a good thing must be better" and increase the "dose" of self-administered therapy. If the program has been correctly prescribed in the first place this can lead only to raised incidence of side-effects without prospect of extra benefit, ultimately undoing any good. The personal setback for the patient can be a disaster for the trial.

These circumstances establish the importance of compliance monitoring. The mainstay procedure in drug trials is pill counting, for which no equivalent exists in physiotherapy. However, motivation is usually accompanied by honesty, and in most cases there is a caregiver to ask as well as the patient.

CONCLUSIONS

The particular problems for clinical trials posed by the nature of physiotherapy, compounded with those of all trials in MND, enforce some major compromises. The most important of these relates to recruitment of control groups, which is impossible to achieve in a way that would be expected of drug trials in other illnesses. Even the basic notions of matched groups and standardized therapies seem incompatible with the combination of physiotherapy and MND. Arguably, the importance of control is limited, given the nature of the illness. If not, trials must fall short of the ideal in this respect. The alternative— resort to single-case studies—offers little assistance to health resource planners who are asked to increase the provision of expensive therapeutic modalities. Other problems may require thoughtful design of physiotherapy trials in MND, but do not appear to be insuperable. Trials of the best possible quality, even if not ideal, are badly needed, because there is much suffering and a potential treatment. The investment of considerable effort in this area is highly worthwhile.

EQUIPMENT

1. Electromyometer. Penny and Giles Transducers Ltd., Airfield Rd., Christchurch, Dorset, England.
2. LIDO (Loredan isokinetic dynamometer). Loredan Biomedical Corporation, 1632 Da Vinci Court, P.O. Box 1154, Davis, Ca. 95617, U.S.A.
3. Cybex 2. Lumex Corporation, Cybex Division, Suite A, 30 Howard Place, Ronkonkoma, N.Y. 11779, U.S.A.
4. Polarised light goniometer. Crane Electronics Ltd., Station Rd., Stoke Golding, Nuneaton, Warwickshire, England.
5. CODA-3 movement monitoring system. Charnwood Dynamics Ltd., 63 Forest Rd., Loughborough, Leicestershire, England.

Acknowledgment: We thank the Motor Neurone Disease Association of Great Britain for their support.

REFERENCES

1. Basmajian JV. Research and retrench. *Phys Ther* 1975;55:607–8.
2. Norris FH, U KS, Denys EH. Amyotrophic lateral sclerosis [Letter]. *Mayo Clin Proc* 1978;53:544.
3. Sinaki M. Rehabilitation. In: Mulder DW, ed. *The diagnosis and treatment of amyotrophic lateral sclerosis: papers from a symposium.* Los Angeles: Houghton Mifflin, 1978:169–93.
4. Frazer FW. Domiciliary physiotherapy — cost and benefit. *Physiotherapy* 1980;662–7.
5. Rose CF. Clinical aspects of motor neuron disease. In: Rose FC, ed. *Motor neuron disease.* London: Pitman, 1977:1–13.
6. Miller RD, Mulder DW, Fowler WS, Olsen AM. Exertional dyspnoea: a primary complaint in unusual cases of progressive muscular atrophy and amyotrophic lateral sclerosis. *Ann Intern Med* 1957;46:119–22.
7. Munsat TL, Andres P, Taft J. The nature of clinical change in amyotrophic lateral sclerosis. In: Tsubaki T, Yase Y, eds. *Amyotrophic lateral sclerosis: recent advances in research and treatment.* Amsterdam: Excerpta Medica, 1988:203–6.
8. Andres PL, Hedlund W, Finison L, Conlon T, Felmus M, Munsat T. Quantitative motor assessment in amyotrophic lateral sclerosis. *Neurology* 1986;36:937–41.

9. Medical Research Council. *Aids to the investigation of peripheral nerve injuries.* War Memorandum (2nd ed.). London: Her Majesty's Stationery Office, 1943.
10. Hyde SA, Scott, OM, Goddard CM. The myometer: the development of a clinical tool. *Physiotherapy* 1983;69:424–7.
11. Thistle HG, Hislop HG, Moffroid M. Isokinetic contraction. A new concept of resistive exercise. *Arch Phys Med Rehab* 1967;48:277–82.
12. Norris FH, Calanchini PR, Fallat RJ, Panchari S, Jewett B. The administration of guanidine in amyotrophic lateral sclerosis. *Neurology* 1974;24:721–8.
13. Hillel AD, Miller RM, McDonald E, Konikow N, Norris FH. Amyotrophic lateral sclerosis severity scale. In: Tsubaki T, Yase Y, eds. *Amyotrophic lateral sclerosis: recent advances in research and treatment.* Amsterdam: Excerpta Medica, 1988:247–52.
14. Rosin AJ. The problems of motor neuron disease. *Age and Ageing* 1976;5:37–42.
15. Newrick PG, Langton-Hewer R. Motor neuron disease: can we do better? A study of 42 patients. *Br Med J* 1984;289:539–42.
16. Williams JI, Physiotherapy is handling. *Physiotherapy* 1986;72:66–7.
17. Bobath B. *Adult hemiplegia: evaluation and treatment.* London: William Heineman, 1978.
18. Chatterton P. Physiotherapy for the terminally ill. *Physiotherapy* 1988;74:42–6.

Amyotrophic Lateral Sclerosis,
edited by F. Clifford Rose.
Demos Publications, New York © 1990.

20

Ethical Issues and Methodological Problems in the Conduct of Clinical Trials in Amyotrophic Lateral Sclerosis

Ian Robinson

Department of Human Sciences, Brunel, The University of West London, Uxbridge, Middlesex, England

The use of randomized controlled trials as the main medium through which putative therapies in amyotrophic lateral sclerosis (ALS) are assessed has produced a series of profound ethical questions. Although many of these questions are not in principle unique to the conduct of trials in relation to ALS, their practical implications for ALS trial design are considerable, not least in terms of the disease process and its effects. Furthermore, the questions cannot be insulated from other methodological issues inherent in trial design and practice. Different kinds of methods employed can raise particular ethical difficulties on the one hand, or provide particular ethical solutions on the other hand. Increasing attention is now being paid to those elements of trial design that minimize ethical problems and maximize ethically optimal objectives.

THE NATURE OF THE BASIC ETHICAL DILEMMA IN CLINICAL TRIALS

At the heart of ethical problems in clinical trials in general, and in particular those in relation to ALS, is the distinction, and potential conflict, between the physician's unique therapeutic obligation to each individual patient, and the scientific duty to seek to expand systematic experimental knowledge for all patients (1). In the first case, the prime, indeed the only, point of reference for the physician is the best interests of the individual patient based on existing clinical knowledge. In the second case, that point of reference is the best interests of all patients — both present and future — toward whom there is an obligation that may both break and transcend the legitimate claims of individual patients to unique therapeutic attention (2). The dilemma can be described in more succinct terms as that between "healer" and "scientist" (3).

Some argue that, in fact, the assumed dilemma or conflict between the "healer" and the "scientist" does not exist because, at any one point of time, the best therapy for any given patient is always that which has received the most current scientific support in properly conducted clinical trials. The results of such trials are — and must be — the foundation of all sound clinical practice (4). Others argue that controlled trials are in any case undertaken only when there is genuine doubt about the best therapeutic agent or clinical course of action, and therefore the appropriate therapeutic strategy applicable to any individual patient can only be determined when relevant trials are concluded and the results are known (5–7). In terms of the doctor's duty of nonmalefeasance ("first, do no harm"), ignorance or even substantial uncertainty about the effects of possible therapies strongly indicate the use of controlled trials. As Perry and Miller argue, "...The physician's obligation to do no harm out of ignorance becomes operative when there is some doubt about the efficacy of an experimental therapy compared with the standard one" (8). From this perspective, all patients who are administered either the test treatment, the best alternative or, if necessary, a placebo, are in a similar, not to say identical, position until the result of the trial is known.

This rather idealized view of the congruity of a physician's therapeutic and scientific obligations has been severely questioned by others who have pointed on the one hand to the array of ethical decisions that are involved at various stages in setting up and running a clinical trial (9,10), and on the other hand pointed to the multiplicity of considerations that may guide clinical practice (11), few of which can be easily reduced to a simple application of the one most scientifically validated therapeutic agent for each patient. In relation to a condition such as ALS, the absence of any such validated therapy emphasizes a range of difficult ethical issues in clinical practice illustrated in the exchange between Carey (12) and Guiloff (13). This situation also reinforces the importance of controlled clinical trials as the primary, perhaps the only, route through which valid and effective therapies might conceivable be derived.

In considering the intersection of ethical and methodological concerns in trial design and execution in relation to ALS, the major issues to be considered in establishing ethically acceptable clinical trial designs have been usefully set out by Schaffner (3). He indicates that ethically informed decisions are particularly important in relation to the following three general issues in the trial process, (a) the initiation of a trial, (b) the selection, allocation, and informed consent of participating patients, and (c) the conduct of the trial and stopping procedures.

In the rest of this analysis these issues are discussed with reference to clinical trials undertaken in relation to ALS and reported in Index Medicus from January 1987 – June 1988, inclusively.

ETHICAL ISSUES IN THE INITIATION OF TRIALS IN ALS

Schaffner argues that one of the main issues in deciding whether a trial of a potential therapeutic agent should be initiated is whether a null hypothesis can reasonably be stated (3). In the case of ALS, at present such a position invariably occurs. Munsat and Brooks note the background to this situation. Over the years, scores of therapeutic trials have been carried out in an attempt either to provide symptomatic relief or to alter the rate of motor neuron loss. No properly controlled and blinded study has ever demonstrated therapeutic efficacy, subjective or objective (14).

In the absence of any treatment alternative other than a placebo, and because of the diversity of etiological arguments brought forward to plausibly explain many different possible treatment paths, it is clearly the case that the efficacy of any new agent is unclear, or unknown. Therefore, in a clinical setting the physician cannot at present recommend any beneficial remedy for ALS, at least not on formal scientific grounds.

A more interesting ethical point in relation to the initiation of a trial in ALS concerns the grounds on which a considerable range of possible therapies have been subject to formal trial assessment. The point here is not so much whether the null hypothesis can be confidently sustained (as it clearly can) but on what grounds one or more of the multitude of possible therapies is chosen for a formal trial. Traditionally, clinical trials on humans have been initiated only after extensive basic research on pathogenesis, and the investigation of the effects of the agent on appropriate animal models. However, as Küther et al., states: "Fragmentary data about the basic pathogenic mechanisms or the lack of appropriate animal models may justify another strategy [to the usual insights from basic research and animal models], especially when a disease is as severe as ALS. Under these circumstances a new hypothesis may arise, from which therapeutic consequences can be deduced directly" (15).

Here the key to the argument is contained in the reference to the severity of the disease. Implicitly, the risks that would be taken in the early testing of a potential therapy for ALS would be greater than those for a disease with a better prognosis. Such risks, at least as far as trial initiation is concerned, largely relate to the skill (and intuition?) with which relevant and testable hypotheses are derived without the benefit of full basic research, and from which in Küther et al.'s words "therapeutic consequences can be deduced directly." This research tactic is one that has potentially problematic consequences. It can be reasonably argued that such a series of scientific short cuts might bring a more immediate, if very slim, chance of alighting on an effective therapeutic agent; on the other hand, such actions may more probably result in a considerable (and ethically dubious) waste of resources in the vast majority of cases because of too-early extrapolation to hypothesis testing in a trial setting. The approach used to overcome the latter problem by a number of clinical investigators is to consider the trial itself as a means of investigating the pathogenesis of the disease. Such strategy is explicitly noted by Mitsumoto et al., who comment: "It is possible that specific treatment will become available only after pathogenesis is discovered, but therapeutic trials could also provide clues to the etiology of this disorder" (16).

A number of trials considered in this analysis have been used in this way, demonstrated, for example, by Brown et al., (17) Dalakis et al., (18), and Kaplan et al., (19), and, indeed, it is hard to locate any trial that does not in its published report comment extensively on the implications of the trial for current pathogenic understanding of the disease. In this way, the gains of the trial are not so much, and perhaps not at all, related to the testing of therapeutic efficacy as in the area of basic understanding about the disease process and its various parameters. In the absence of any major therapeutic advance, such gains are welcome but they raise special ethical issues, unless participating patients are fully informed that this objective is one, or the major, aim in initiating the trial. If patients are not so informed, the ethical risk is that the hopes of patients may be unjustifiably raised that therapeutic rewards would be likely to arise from such trials.

It may be that the direct and indirect pressures from patients themselves to initiate formal testing of therapeutic agents in a condition such as ALS, as well as the overall dynamics of clinical research itself, both increase the probability that the scientific short-circuit route to trials will be adopted. The hypothesis – therapeutic deduction route mapped out by Küther could lead to premature testing of possible drug therapies based on extrapolations from well-known, but incomplete, animal models, or from inferences from other broadly similar disease profiles. A similar pattern can be seen occurring in response to patient-reported benefits from drugs or other therapies. Some have suggested that reports of any therapeutic benefit are so uncommon in ALS that careful attention should be paid to any agent so implicated (14) from whatever source; the moral dilemma facing the researcher is the possibility, however remote, that a potential therapy may indeed prove beneficial despite considerable scientific skepticism as to the rationale for the imputed benefit. Norris et al., (20), in a brief account of a trial of octanosol in ALS, indicate that the major (and only stated) initiating factor in the trial was a sequence of reports from patients, and the ALS Society of America indicating perceived benefits. The possibility of such reports reflecting real means of alleviating ALS could not easily be dismissed in view of the absence of an agreed etiology for ALS, and the need to be responsive to widespread claims of beneficial effects, but establishing a trial in these circumstances reduces the usual scientific threshold at which a potential therapeutic agent would be expected to be subject to formal trial test, with, at least in scientific terms, a lower chance of success in producing positive results.

There are other consequences of initiating a wide range of trials in ALS. First, the majority of such trials are too small, frequently with less than 10 patients being used. This small size appears to be related to uncertainty over the therapeutic status of the agent, the difficulty of obtaining larger numbers of patients on the specified trial criteria, practical problems in administering the drug and therapy concerned, or problems in obtaining resources both financial and professional to undertake a larger trial. When such trials are of phase I status and are mainly concerned with establishing toxicity and dosage, small numbers of patients are relatively unproblematic, but conclusive inferences should not be drawn about the possible therapeutic status of the agent because they cannot be made on a sound statistical basis, particularly because only the grossest changes are likely to be assessable with any confidence. Such a situation may have occurred with trials involving plasmapheresis in ALS in which, during a period of several years after Patten's small trial on three patients (21), other small trials by Shy et al., Olarte et al. (23), and Keleman et al. (24), were carried out after which Rudnicki et al. (25) suggested a negligible role for the treatment in changing the course of the disease. This conclusion may indeed be proved right, but it is difficult on the basis of these trials to state on firm statistical grounds that this is indeed the case. Without a formal and blinded control group and when baseline data from a small number of patients — or hypothetical extrapolations of them — are used as the standard against which possible beneficial changes are measured, firm observations of the statistical absence (as well as occasionally the presence) of positive changes are incautious. One danger in initiating only, or mainly, small trials in ALS is that they may not allow the formal registration of the subtle changes that have been argued to be the most likely to be the first demonstrated effect of a useful therapy (14). Undoubtedly, the absence of measured beneficial changes in many of the small trials initiated properly indicates the lack of efficacy of a potential therapy. On formal statistical grounds it could convincingly be argued that larger trials are needed to uncover marginal — but still — important changes that might have been below the statistical power of a small trial to detect with any realistic degree of confidence.

The statistical power of many of the smaller trials in ALS, even when they are of phase II or III status, is such that only total disease arrest, or a very substantial change in the expected course of the disease, could be detected with high confidence limits. Munsat and Brooks make this point in their commentary on the trials of Mitsumoto et al. (26), Caroscio et al. (27), and Brooke et al. (28) on the effect of thyrotropin-releasing hormone (TRH) in ALS. They note in particular in relation to the study of Brooke et al. that "The authors rightly point out that their study was designed to have a 95% chance of finding a total arrest of the disease process and an 84% chance of finding an 80% reduction in the rate of deterioration of ALS. Unfortunately, such strict criteria may preclude recognition of a less dramatic effect" (14) and further that ". . . We must be aware that the first step in treating this disease may be small. . . If we construct too rigid criteria for the initial evaluation of a drug, we will have the self-fulfilling prophecy of finding no treatment for the disease. . . Small steps in sequence may provide the answer to effective therapy."

Munsat and Brooks seem to be indicating, and there is at least circumstantial evidence for this point, that the overwhelmingly bad short-term prognosis for patients with ALS has persuaded clinical researchers implicitly to set their own objectives equally high in the same short term. Thus, some trials appear to be initiated and statistically assessed as though the sole aim is the immediate conquest of the complete disease process, rather than a recognition of the often slow, hesitant, and partial progress to this end; at least this is the net effect of the stringent statistical criteria on which Munsat and Brooks comment. Brooke replies to the discussion by indicating that such stringency is a necessary component of trials (especially of TRH) in which expectations are high and the hopes of patients have been prematurely raised (29). Mitsumoto and colleagues do, however, acknowledge that it is possible that they may have missed subtle benefits in their trial, and suggest that the methodological approach to such clinical trials needs reevaluation (30). Other investigators have expressed similar reservations about the ability of their trial procedures to locate modest beneficial effects (31,32).

The key point is that such trials are not undertaken out of idle scientific curiosity, but in the knowledge of the high stakes that both the profession and patients have in their outcome. In this respect, it is interesting to consider the conduct of trials with reference to the distinction made by the social scientist Max Weber between research being "value relevant" but at the same time being "value free," (33), i.e., trials could be *initiated* on the basis of their importance and salience to the objectives of patients, physicians, and scientists involved, i.e., trials are relevant to their values, but the *conduct* of the trials is undertaken in a value free or scientific way. The difficulty lies in separating these two elements. Scientists, and clinicians as well as patients, can quickly come to have substantial personal interests in the running and outcome as well as the initiation of trials, however hard they try to suspend individual interests and values in the face of discordant scientific information. There is ultimately a fine line between the disinterested but determinedly dogged pursuit of scientific truth about a potential therapy, and the continual and fruitless personal commitment to research and trials on a therapy whose efficacy has not, and arguably never will be, scientifically proven. Radically changing lines of inquiry and developing new initiatives — however much it may be demanded by the tenets of scientific investigation — is a costly process. In summary, in this process there are two equal and opposite ethical and scientific dangers. The first results from overcommitment to evaluating one particular potential therapy beyond the point where on scientific grounds that commitment is rewarding, and the simultaneous and corresponding rejection of other lines of inquiry. The second results from, if anything, a scientific undercommitment to the evaluation of any one therapy as a multiplicity of potential agents are tested in small trials, without the necessary scientific attention to possible marginal but beneficial effects of the agent, which might be more statistically evident (or would be more conclusively disproven) in larger and longer trials.

SELECTION, ALLOCATION, AND INFORMED CONSENT OF PARTICIPATING PATIENTS

The selection of patients for trials in ALS is a special problem. The relatively low incidence of the disease, the relatively swift physical trajectory it often takes, and the range of functions quickly affected in major ways pose considerable difficulties. The initial location of sufficient ALS patients is a problem of some magnitude for trials in small centers. The selection criteria for entry into a trial focuses attention on some essential requirements, which must include a secure diagnosis as well as an effective system of of grading and measuring the disease ands its effects , both on an inter- and intrapatient basis, which should be reasonably confidently compared across different trials in different settings and different countries. Neither of these issues are trivial. As far as a secure diagnosis is concerned, as Mitsumoto et al. notes, despite a recognition that "The diagnosis of ALS is made with surprising uniformity by physicians.... the clinical limits of ALS have not been well defined" (16). In relation to the assessment of disease state, measures such as the Norris scale (34), widely used and regarded as a helpful addition to the repertory of assessments of ALS, have been argued to need supplementation for more precise investigation of subtle disease changes (16), but there are further problems that revolve around the course of the disease and its consequences for trial design. Some of these are referred to by Küther et al. (15). With severely affected patients it is necessary to ensure, as far as possible, that survival time is expected to be beyond the end of the trial, perhaps on the basis of pulmonary function at entry. In longer trials, which may be necessary for the effective testing of some drugs, this requirement could lead to relatively atypical cases of ALS being used. There is also the implication by Küther et al. that constellations of atypical long-term survivors in particular clinical centers could be used for a range of trials and thereby introduce systematic, but unintended, biases in research findings. In a more general sense, patient selection may also be used to explain the discrepancy between two different trials, as between those of de Jong et al. (35) and Küther and Struppler (36) on *N*-acetylcysteine. In this respect, the source of patients, the type of drug under test, and the duration of the trial may give rise to quite discrepant sets of participating patients even within what superficially appears to be a broadly similar disease profile.

The severity of the disease, or particular functions associated with it, both at the outset of, and during, the trial, may be an especially important factor in realistically assessing the benefits of therapy. in relation to serious neuromuscular diseases, the loss of neural function at the point of test of the drug may be so great that it would be extraordinary to expect any significant regeneration of tissue or function. The "typical" ALS patient used in a trial setting could be so advanced in the loss of motor neurons that it may be clinically unrealistic to expect major or even minor positive and fundamental regenerative effects to occur from therapy. On the other hand, to include patients earlier in the disease process may give rise to diagnostic uncertainties, as well as lead to the use of cases whose prognosis is unclear and difficult to measure. Küther et al. express the point thus: "... It has to be noted that ALS patients with unequivocal symptoms are often in an advanced state of their disease with a considerable amount of motor neurons lost. Although these patients may be best suited for clinical measurements, the efficacy even of an optimal therapy may be rather limited. It can be assumed that the beneficial effect of a tested agent in a degenerative disease may be most pronounced in preclinical or initial stages, when the bulk of motor neurons are still intact. These patients, however, introduce much uncertainty with respect to their further progression, so that it seems virtually impossible to test a treatment in this group" (15).

This point can be further refined to suggest that there might be a particular phase of the disease that would be more susceptible to modification than any other phase. In reviewing studies of TRH in ALS one account noted that "The lack of clear-cut effects has been attributed to a therapeutic window; that is, beneficial effects may not be seen if doses were either too high or too low, or if the patient was examined too soon or too late" (37).

The committee responsible for this observation was skeptical that the lack of consistent effects of the drug could be explained in this way, but nonetheless there are grounds for believing that not all points in a trajectory of neurological deterioration are equally amenable to therapeutic attention.

A further point relates especially to the ethical context of patient selection. The willingness of patients to participate in any trial with a condition such as ALS, almost whatever its design, is substantial. There is some evidence that even this substantial willingness increases with the progression of serious conditions such as ALS. For the patient, perhaps as for the clinician–researcher, the ratio of cost and benefits of trial participation weighs increasingly heavily in favor of the benefits. Although the chances of any positive results in slowing or stopping the disease process may be very small, set against the fatal course of ALS, even such a slim possibility is a potential bonus. The benefits perceived by patients are thus most likely to be interestedly personal, rather than disinterestedly scientific. In this situation there is clearly additional pressure on the trial scientist to accept severely affected patients into the trial as much for an extension of the medical "healing" as for the medical "scientific" role. The trial in this setting could thus become de facto an extension of clinical support by other means. This pressure to participate and its likely resolution could itself compound the problems of using more severely affected patients in ALS trials.

Some of the ethical issues related to patient selection are also relevant to the process of randomization. Although many of the trials considered in this analysis are not randomized, partly because of the nature of the trial and trial size, but also because of other unclear considerations, randomization in a more formal assessment of therapeutic effect is important, and is regarded by many investigators as essential (38–41). Knowing that in the current state of scientific knowledge the alternative (control) therapy to the treatment under trial is almost certain to be a placebo, there is considerable additional pressure by each patient to be placed in the treatment group. Only the most rigorous randomization process can counter the possible (indeed probable) biases inherent in any other system of patient allocation, yet the process of randomization itself has been argued to have as many significant ethical drawbacks as it has scientific advantages. Some of these dilemmas have recently been reconsidered in the light of substantial difficulties in recruitment to trials of therapies for various cancers (42). The most difficult ethical problem raised about randomization and the scientifically sound allocation of patients to the appropriate arms of a trial protocol is the implication for the clinical care of the participating patients (43). Although in the case of ALS there is not even minimally effective alternative therapy and thus no question of denying patients access to it through randomization, it is still conceivable that the best clinical care in the broadest sense might be compromised by such randomization. Such problems posed to clinical care might include constraints on the most appropriate administration of the complete range of drugs of choice for symptomatic relief, perhaps inhibitions to the institution of active measures to enhance pulmonary function in the later stages of the disease, and a lessening of the more general ability to radically change clinical strategy if the circumstances dictated it. Apart from the ethical consequences for physicians' own perception of their proper duties to their patients through their healing or scientific role, randomization also poses questions about how the properly informed consent of patients to a trial can, or should, be obtained.

The question of informed consent by patients in clinical trials is complex. Almost more has been written about the question of informed consent than any other issue in trial design. Many writers agree that the question of informed consent by patients participating in trials is in principle an ethically almost irresolvable problem (44–46). This is because of the formal difficulty of identifying for every patient what constitutes appropriate "information" on which consent might legitimately be based, and in turn what constitutes "consent." In trial practice, various pragmatic solutions to these issues have been adopted to ensure that trials can proceed with a minimum of ethical concern — regularly formalized under the direction of ethics committees or institutional review boards. In the case of those with ALS, a series of ethical difficulties may arise in seeking informed consent. Some of these are technically soluble, for example, such as those that result from a functional inability to sign written consent forms. Others relate to the more fundamental difficulties indicated that arise from ambiguity and lack of clarity over what constitutes "consent" and "being informed."

There is, and perhaps has to be, a general assumption in relation to the general objectives of trials that the interests of patients and those of clinicians and medical scientists are similar, if not identical. If this is the case, then the ethical issues posed by the question of informed consent are less problematic, but Schaffner indicates that although physicians may quite reasonably act on this basis, patients may have quite rationally different preferences about their objectives in respect of trials (3). For example, Fried argues that "Even in medically equivalent cases, patients may have quite different value systems: their life plans may have quite different structures. And though the overall prognosis, the overall expected value of the therapies may be practically the same, the composition of the risks and benefits of the therapy might be different" (47). These potentially different objectives may not easily become visible because of the degree of passivity the patient is normally expected to assume in a trial setting; indeed such passivity can be seen in some ways as integral to the exercise of strict scientific control in the trial protocol. The patient is not generally considered to be an active participant in the trial process, except to originally consent to be part of the trial, and to arrange to be available for treatments or assessments as required.

In the debate about the degree of information required to properly obtain informed consent, there are two contrasting views. The first is that the minimum necessary information should be given, particularly about randomization because this could seriously affect participation, and perhaps make some trials impossible (48). The other and opposing perspective is that not only should as complete information as possible be given to potential participants, but that they should in some real sense become partners in the trial. In this process the patient ". . . elects to become a subject in the trial, thereby allowing the physician to assign a protocol-dictated treatment rather than an individualised treatment. In one view the patient [thus] elects to become a co-adventurer in the search for new knowledge rather than a mere object of scrutiny" (49). This role of the patient – as partner – overcomes some of the possible problems centered on randomization (1), and also reduces the conflict between the healing and scientific aspects of the physician-investigator's role; but this view rests in part on the existence of a strong altruistic, rather than totally self-interested, component among patients' objectives. In other words, the assumption is that many patients would be prepared to participate for the furtherance of scientific knowledge for other (future) patients, not only for their own benefit. There is almost no formal and systematic research on what patients' — as opposed to physicians' or scientists' — objectives are in relation to their participation in trials. What little data exist show that there is indeed a considerable altruistic element in such participation, even alongside substantial self-interest (50,51). As already indicated, the willingness of patients to participate in trials for ALS is considerable, so that the question of what information is realistically required to obtain informed consent in this situation is a complex one; unless the minimalist view is taken (48), the information given should include that indicated in the Nuremberg Code: ". . . the nature, duration and purpose of the experiment, the method and means by which it is conducted, all inconveniences and hazards reasonably to be expected, and the effects upon his health or person which may possibly come from his participation. . . " (52).

One of the most important factors may be that associated with "inconveniences and hazards." Although those with ALS have a poor prognosis, and thus may be less subjectively influenced by such issues, this perspective really fails to take account the complexity of the quality of life. To those severely affected by ALS, the imposition of possible — perhaps even likely — side-effects of such techniques as plasmapheresis or the administration of interferon by various methods is a major problem. Even medically marginal, but personally problematic side-effects superimposed on a rapidly declining physical condition can undermine a modest quality of life. Here the equation for the patient may well be between the unpredictable but possible benefits of the treatment, set against the generally more predictable side-effects. In patients with ALS, the crucial information necessary for adequate consent could be that related to the medical hazards associated with the trial design.

CONDUCT OF THE TRIAL AND STOPPING PROCEDURES

There are a series of issues that interweave ethical and methodological problems in the conduct and stopping of trials of drugs for ALS. These range from the problems associated with continuous assessment of change in such trials, to the ability to achieve true blinding, given the often clinically visible effects of drug therapies, through the practical management of seriously ill patients in a trial setting, to the criteria on which a trial should be stopped.

The question of what should be assessed and how that assessment should be undertaken is a particularly difficult issue. Apart from the difficulties of measurement per se and of obtaining an agreed valid, reliable, and widely used system, the issue is to what extent trials should be concerned with the precise measurement of motor neuron loss and possible regeneration, or be concerned with functional changes that may or may not be correlated with such loss or regeneration. This debate is one that permeates the trial process, and also relates to the question of the extent to which trials should be concerned with a further exploration of pathogenesis as well as therapeutic efficacy at a functional level. This leads on to a further issue about the status of objective measurements (whether fundamental or functional in emphasis) in relation to subjective indicators of improvement.

The question is: To what extent should credibility be attached to such subjective indicators that may be associated with the patients' perception of the quality of their lives, although not necessarily associated with any ascertainable signs of objective improvement? A number of trials have noted such subjective indications of improvement, e.g., a study of TRH in an early trial (53), and in a range of other trials (54,55). One school of thought is that such subjective indicators have little place in trials of ALS, whereas another is that they must be taken seriously, particularly if related to therapeutic measures in a controlled trial, because of the dearth of positive effects of any kind noted in such trials. In this regard, it has been argued that subjective indicators can in fact more profitably be used than is commonly assumed (56) and that in any case, the ability to marginally improve a patient's perceived quality of life is of some substance.

The question of whether a trial of many of the therapies tested in relation to ALS can be truly blind is a serious issue. It is almost impossible to maintain blinding in certain cases even with randomization and the most stringent precautions. The effects (and/or side-effects) of some drugs are so clear, either to the patient or to the supervising physician, and so dissimilar to any realistic placebo, it is unlikely that the blinding can be maintained. This has been discussed, particularly in relation to trials of TRH because, as one of the few substances demonstrated in studies to have some, albeit very temporary effect, the circumstances in which this effect came to be identified is of considerable importance (37). As the Committee on Health Care Issues indicates, "One of the difficulties in using TRH and in performing a double-blind trial is that the side effects are obvious to both patient and examiner." In one of the trials on TRH such a problem is also commented on by Brooks (32). After noting that "The increased number of responses [occurring] concurrently with identical autonomic effects of TRH . . . have caused concern among many investigators because they make true blinding of the patient to TRH administration difficult," he then goes on to argue that "no severe autonomic side effects" were noted in the TRH group in his study. Guiloff and colleagues (55) make a similar point in their trial of a TRH analogue. "The double-blind nature of the trial may be questioned because of the side effects of the drug. However, in 50% of the patients they were not clinically significant and a few patients had side effects with placebo (nausea, vomiting). Measurements that showed the most clear drug effect (speech, respiration) are unlikely to have had observer bias . . ."

The problem is that the effects do not necessarily have to be severe for the blinding to be undone. Research in other trials not on ALS has shown how remarkably fragile blinding procedures are (57), and it is possible that this fact may have created inhibiting difficulties for more extensive trials of some substances.

The practical management of participating patients, often with major functional problems, in a trial setting is likely to be particularly difficult. Their continued participation, as opposed to their initial agreement to be involved in the trial, may be contingent on the personal rewards (in terms of therapeutic benefit) they perceive in the trial situation. for example, in the trial by Mora et al. of interferon in ALS it is reported that 4 of 10 patients withdrew during the trial because they felt no apparent benefit (58). Although it may not be so easy to identify other related factors associated with such withdrawals, the combination of severely affected patients, frequent (and perhaps continuous) need for hospitalization during the trial, and substantial side-effects are likely to be among the most important. Withdrawals of patients are not an unexpected occurrence in trials, but because the number of original participants in many ALS trials is so small, any decrease in numbers is a serious loss and will seriously affect the assessment of trial results. These points must be considered in relation to the type and motivation of patients participating in trials, and leads back to the issue of patient selection discussed above.

The rules of stopping have exercised many concerned with the ethical and statistical aspects of trial design (59–61) and is particularly apposite in relation to ALS trials. The key objective of a trial design with good stopping rules is to maximize the degree of confidence with which the effects under study (negative or positive) are detected as quickly as possible. This enables those in the less favored arm of a trial to receive that treatment (placebo or active therapy) for as little time as possible. Conventional trial designs, without crossover, that are still widely used in relation to trials in ALS may provide an appropriate and scientifically satisfactory evaluation of the drugs under test if appropriate statistical procedures are employed in relation to specified objectives, but they have considerable ethical drawbacks, which relate partly to the question of initial randomization and its implications for those receiving what may be thought to be the less clinically favored treatment (or no treatment in the case of a placebo being used), and partly to the concept of a single stopping point that occurs when the treatment odds in favor of one arm of the trial have become clearer and therefore even more disadvantageous to either the treatment or the control group.

The majority of clinical trials in relation to ALS follow this conventional trial design, insofar as control groups are used, but the issue has not been so much that patients in one trial arm have failed to receive what proved to be the more beneficial treatment accorded to others, but that they were exposed to a treatment that produced significantly more side-effects than its alternative (usually a placebo) did. In ethical terms the two situations are comparable. In this setting, the major ameliorating factor is the extent to which the trial has led to a gain of scientific knowledge about the disease process, about which objective the participating patients were already fully informed, and in relation to which they had given their consent.

Nonetheless in phase II and particularly in phase III trials there are other modifications of the basic trial technique that produce significantly greater ethical advantages. A crossover technique produces a situation that is ethically more acceptable, although it still has the disadvantages of relatively long exposure for all patients to a treatment regime that will come to be statistically relegated in favor of another (62). In view of these problems, a great number of alternatives have been suggested that attempt to minimize the number of patients, and the length of time they spend in treatment situations subsequently found to be without benefit.

Sequential or adaptive designs were one of the first serious attempts to deal with these problematic ethical issues (63), because they allow for the minimum number of patients to be in what is proving to be the least effective track of the trial as it progressed. Even so, ethical objections could still be levied against such designs because of the initial randomization that involved scientific, rather than clinical, decisions about the placing of participating patients. For this reason, there has been a revival of interest in Bayesian-based trial designs, which seek to maximize the extent to which clinical criteria about patient care could be applied even in a trial situation (64–66). Such trial designs comprise two main elements. First is the pooling of expert judgments on the best treatment track for individual participating patients where they are allocated to the appropriate trial arms, based on a probabilistic model. The underlying philosophy might be described as the arms of the trial being allocated to the patients rather than the patients being allocated to the arms. The second element is a continuous monitoring of changing expert opinions as a result of which allocations are modified substantially in favor of more favored treatment strategies. This procedure is controversial because randomization in its commonly understood sense is not employed, but it has very substantial ethical virtues in relation to what is a very difficult ethical problem (62). In the case of the present knowledge of ALS, the virtues of this approach would not lie so much in more ethical allocations to therapeutic trials with two competitive and potentially beneficial therapies, but would allow the appropriate differential allocation of patients to trials in which at least one of the agents under test was as likely to produce potent side-effects as to be potentially beneficial. Combined with the interesting and less problematic stopping rules proposed by Meier (9), such a trial design may have considerable advantages over more traditional designs.

Finally, given some of the problems enumerated above in creating both an ethically acceptable and scientifically sound trial in ALS, two other strategies may be employed that have recently been argued to have special virtues. Of particular interest is the possibility of randomized trials in individual patients. In a review article, Guyatt et al. (67) argue that such a strategy is apposite in circumstances in which extrapolation from existing clinical trials to individual patients is problematic, when problems exist in accumulating sufficient patients for a trial, or indeed when a formal trial has yet to be undertaken. All of these situations may obtain in relation to ALS. Essentially, as Guyatt et al. argue, the single-person (N = 1) trial is where treatment modalities are systematically varied over a series of periods in a single individual. Using procedures similar to normal crossover designs, a careful evaluation can be undertaken of the extent to which a sequenced series of treatments (blind to both the patient and physician) affect the disease course (68,69). Although such trials must be seen as related to the patient under trial and not to all such patients, a body of useful data may be accumulated that, if carefully analyzed, would stand comparison with much data gained from other small and perhaps inadequately statistically monitored trials. This trial design has the very considerable ethical advantage that it can be considered to combine clinical care with an experimental approach, and thereby overcome some of the relatively intractable conflicts of ethical interest previously discussed.

In relation to the ex-post-facto assessment of a series of small trials in ALS, the use of meta-analysis may prove of some importance. Meta-analysis is a procedure for analyzing and combining the results of previous trials. Sacks et al. (70) argue that this kind of analysis allows an increase in statistical power for primary end-points; can be used to resolve uncertainty when reports disagree, can improve estimates of effect size, and can answer questions that may not have been posed at the trial outset. The majority of such analyses have been undertaken since 1980 (70). The key to the effectiveness of such analyses depends on the extent to which acceptable criteria can be established on which trials might be combined for statistical purposes. In the case of ALS combinations of small trials, in relation to TRH and possibly interferon and plasmapheresis, may be amenable to attention through this medium, although one of the major difficulties is the extent to which control groups, randomization, and blinding procedures have been commonly applied. With the particular problems associated with establishing viable trials in ALS, the use of meta-analysis suggests that a further potentially profitable route of trial assessment could be established.

CONCLUSIONS

There is a considerable range of ethical problems generated in the course of ALS trials, which are intricately interwoven with methodological issues. Although many of these problems are inherent in overall trial design rather than specifically located in the formal testing of potential therapies in ALS, the nature of the disease and the special pressures it generates among patients and investigating clinicians raise particular difficulties. These special pressures arise in the process of initiating trials; in the selection, allocation, and informed consent of participating patients; and in trial conduct and the stopping rules employed.

A large number, perhaps too many, small trials are being conducted without the necessary statistical power to detect potentially modest changes in the functional status of the patient or in the disease process itself. The selection of participating patients, as well as the accurate measurement of their disease status, have not been undertaken on a sufficiently consistent or appropriate basis to confidently make clear assessments on a comparative basis. The ability to genuinely blind controlled trials in ALS is an additional cause of major concern, as is the extent to which a combination of severely affected patients and frequent, major side-effects in some trials produce problems of trial management. The stopping rules of trials, particularly in the context of the ethical consequences of randomization, need further examination and it was suggested that Bayesian-influenced trial designs may have some virtues in this respect. Two additional strategies — single-person trials and meta-analyses — may allow expansion of the ways in which some of the more difficult ethical and methodological issues in ALS trial design can be overcome or compensated for.

REFERENCES

1. Gifford F. The conflict between randomised clinical trials and the therapeutic obligation. *J Med Philos* 1986;11:347–66.
2. Clayton D. Ethically optimised designs. *Br J Clin Pharmacol* 1982;13:469–80.
3. Schaffner KF. Ethical problems in clinical trials. *J Med Philos* 1986;11:297–316.
4. Ditchley Foundation report. The scientific and ethical basis of the clinical evaluation of medicines. *Eur J Clin Pharmacol* 1980;18:129–34.
5. Byar DP, Simon RN, Friedewald WT, et al. Randomised clinical trials. *N Engl J Med* 1976;74:295.
6. Giertz G. Ethics of randomised trials. *J Med Ethics* 1980;6:55.
7. Schafer A. The ethics of the randomised clinical trial. *N Engl J Med* 1982;307:719.
8. Perry CB, Miller ST. Ethical consideration of clinical research. *J Am Geriat Soc* 1986;34:49–51.
9. Meier P. Terminating a trial — the ethical problem. *Clin Pharmacol Ther* 1979;25:637–40.
10. Burkhardt R, Kienle G. Basic problems in controlled clinical trials. *J Med Ethics* 1983;9:80–4.
11. Leigh H, Reiser MF. *The patient.* New York: Plenum Medical, 1980. Motor neuron disease — a challenge to medical ethics. *J R Soc Med* 1986;79:216–20.
12. Carey JS. Motor neuron disease and ethics: a neurologist's point of view. J R Soc Med 1986;79:216 20.
13. Guiloff RJ. Motor neuron disease and ethics: a neurologist's point of view. *J R Soc Med* 1987;80:473–4.
14. Munsat TL, Brooks BR. Don't throw the baby out with the bathwater (Letter) *Neurology* 1987;37:544–5.
15. Küther G, Struppler A, Lipinski HG. Therapeutic trials in ALS. In: Cosi V, Kato AC, Parlette W, Pinelli P, Poloni M, eds. *Amyotrophic lateral sclerosis— therapeutic, psychological and research aspects.* 1986:355.
16. Mitsumoto H, Hanson MR, Chad DA. Amyotrophic lateral sclerosis: recent advances in pathogenesis and clinical trials. *Arch Neurol* 1988;45:189–202.
17. Brown RH, Hauser SL, Harrington H, Weiner HL. Failure of immunosuppression with a ten to fourteen day course of high dose intravenous cyclophosphamide to alter the progression of amyotrophic lateral sclerosis. *Arch Neurol* 1986;43:383–4.
18. Dalakis MC, Aksamit AJ, Madden DL, Sever JL. Administration of recombinant human leucocyte (alpha) 2-interferon in patients with amyotrophic lateral sclerosis. *Arch Neurol* 1986;43:933–5.
19. Kaplan MM, Taft JA, Reichlin S, Munsat TL. Sustained rises in serum thyrotropin, thyroxine and triiodothyronine during long-term continuous thyrotropin-releasing hormone treatment in patients with amyotrophic lateral sclerosis. *J Clin Endocrinol Metabol* 1986;63:808–14.
20. Norris F, Denys EH, Fallat RJ. Trial of octonasol in amyotrophic lateral sclerosis. *Neurology* 1986;36:1263–4.
21. Patten BM. Neuropathy and motor neuron syndromes associated with plasma cell disease. *Acta Neurol Scand* 1984;69:47–61.
22. Shy ME, Trojaborg W, Smith T, et al. Motor neuron disease and plasma cell dyscrasia. *Neurology* 1985;35(Suppl 1):107.

23. Olarte MR, Schoenfeldt R, McKiernan G, Rowland LP. Plasmapheresis in amyotrophic lateral sclerosis. *Ann Neurol* 1980;8:644–5.
24. Keleman J, Hedlund W, Orlin JB, Berkman EM, Munsat TL, Plasmapheresis with immunosuppression in amyotrophic lateral sclerosis. *Arch Neurol* 1983;40:752–3.
25. Rudnicki S, Chad DA, Drachman DA, Smith TW, Anwer UE, Levitan N. Motor neuron disease and paraproteinemia. *Neurology* 1987;37:335–7.
26. Mitsumoto H, Salgado ED, Negroski D, et al. Amyotrophic lateral sclerosis: effects of acute intravenous and chronic subcutaneous administration of thyrotropin-releasing hormone in controlled trials *Neurology* 1986,36:152–9.
27. Caroscio JT, Cohen JA, Zawodniak J, et al. A double-blind placebo controlled study of TRH in amyotrophic lateral sclerosis. *Neurology* 1986;36:141–5.
28. Brooke MH, Florence JM, Heller SL, et al. Controlled trial of thyrotropin-releasing hormone in amyotrophic lateral sclerosis. *Neurology* 1986;36:146–51.
29. Brooke MH. Reply to Munsat and Brooks [Letter]. *Neurology* 1987;37:545.
30. Mitsumoto H, Hanson MR, Salanga VD. Reply to Munsat and Brooks [Letter]. *Neurology* 1987;37:545.
31. Hawley RJ, Kratz R, Goodman RR, McCutchen CB, Sirdofsky M, Hanson PA. Treatment of amyotrophic lateral sclerosis with the TRH analog DN-1417. *Neurology* 1987;37:715–7.
32. Brooks BR, Sufit RL, Montgomery GK, Beaulieu DA, Erickson LM. Intravenous thyrotropin-releasing hormone in patients with amyotrophic lateral sclerosis. *Neurol Clin* 1987;5:143–58.
33. Giddens A. *Politics and sociology in the thought of Max Weber.* London: Macmillan, 1972.
34. Norris FH, Calanchini PR, Fallat RJ, et al. The administration of guanidine in amyotrophic lateral sclerosis. *Neurology* 1974;24:721–8.
35. de Jong JMBV, den Hartog Jager WA, Vyth A, Timmer JG. Attepted treatment of motor neuron disease with N-acetylcysteine and dithiothreitol. In: Cosi V, Kato AC, Parlette W, Pinelli P, Poloni M, eds. *Amyotrophic lateral sclerosis— therapeutic, psychological and and research aspects.* New York: Plenum Press, 1986.
36. Kuther G, Struppler A. Therapeutic trial with *N*-acetylcysteine in amyotrophic lateral sclerosis. In: Cosi V, Kato AC, Parlette W, Pinelli P, Poloni M, eds. *Amyotrophic lateral sclerosis— therapeutic, psychological and research aspects.* New York: Plenum Press, 1986.
37. Committe on Health Care Issues. American Neurological Association. Current status of thyrotropin-releasing hormone therapy in amyotrophic lateral sclerosis. *Ann Neurol* 1987;22:541–3.
38. Armitage P. The role of randomisation in clinical trials. *Stat Med* 1982;1:345–52.
39. Spodick DH. The randomised controlled clinical trial: scientific and ethical bases. *Am J Med* 1983;73:420–5.
40. Waldenstrom J. The ethics of randomisation. *Prog Clin Biol Res* 1983;128:243–9..
41. Moser M. Randomised clinical trials: problems and values. *Am J Emerg Med* 1986;4:173–8.
42. Brahams D. Randomised trials and informed consent. *Lancet* 1988;2:1033–4.
43. Marquis D. An argument that all prerandomised trials are unethical *J Med Phil* 1986;11:367–84.
44. Levine RJ. The apparent incompatibility between informed consent and placebo-controlled clinical trials *Clin Pharmacol Ther* 1987;42:247–56.

45. Kopelman L. Consent and randomised clinical trials: are there moral or design problems? *J Med Philos* 1986;11:317–46.
46. Kirby MD. Informed consent? What does it mean? *J Med Ethics* 1983;9:69–75.
47. Fried C. *Medical experimentation: personal integrity and social policy.* New York: American Elsevier.
48. Baum M. Do we need informed consent? *Lancet* 1986;2:911–2.
49. Coulehan JL, Schaffner KF, Block M. Ethics of clinical trials in family medecine. *J Fam Pract* 1985;21:217–22.
50. Saurbrey N, Jensen J. Elmegaard Rasmussen P, Gjorup T, Guldager H, Rilis P. Danish patients' attitudes to scientific-ethical questions: an interview study focusing on therapeutic trials. *Acta Med Scan* 1984;215:99–104.
51. Wynne A. Effects and benefits: the evaluation of hyperbaric oxygen as a therapy by participants in a clinical trial. Academic working paper. London: Brunel-Arms Research Unit, Brunel University, 1988.
52. The Nuremberg Code. Trials of war criminals before Nuremberg military tribunals under council law no. 10. *Medical Case* 1947;2:181–3.
53. Engel WK. Siddique T, Nocoloff JT. Effect on weakness and spasticity in amyotrophic lateral sclerosis of thyrotropin-releasing hormone. *Lancet* 1985;2:73–5.
54. Provinciali L, Giovanoli AR, Di Bella P, Baroni M, Dellantonio R. A therapeutic trial of a thymic factor in amyotrophic lateral sclerosis. In: Cosi V, Kato AC, Parlette W, Pinelli P, Poloni M, eds. *Amyotrophic lateral sclerosis— therapeutic, psychological and research aspects.* 1986.
55. Guiloff RJ, Eckland DJA, Demaine C, Hoare RC, Macrae KD, Lightman SL. Controlled acute trial of a thyrotropin-releasing hormone analogue (RX77368) in motor neuron disease. *J Neurol Neurosurg Psychiatry* 1987;50:1359–70.
56. Robinson I. Analysing the structure of 23 clinical trials in multiple sclerosis. *Neuroepidemiology* 1987;6:46–76.
57. Stallone F, Mendlewicz J, Fieve RR. How blind is double blind? An assessment in the study of lithium prophylaxis. *Psychol Med* 1976;5:78–82.
58. Mora JS, Munsat TL, Kao KP, et al. Intrathecal administration of natural human interferon alpha in amyotrophic lateral sclerosis. *Neurology* 1986;36:1137–40.
59. Zelen M. The randomisation and stratification of patients to clinical trials. *J Chron Dis* 1974;27:365–75.
60. Zelen M. A new design for randomised clinical trials. *N Engl J Med* 1979;300:1242–5.
61. Pocock SJ. *Clinical trials: a practical approach.* London: Wiley 1983.
62. Kadane JB. Progress towards a more ethical method for clinical trials. *J Med Philos* 1986;11:385–404.
63. Armitage P. Sequential medical trials. Oxford: Blacwell Publications, 1975.
64. Kadane J, Sedransk N. towards a more ethical clinical trial. In: Bernado et al. *Bayesian statistics.* Valencia University of Valencia, 1980:326.
65. Sedransk N. Allocation of sequentially available units to treatment groups. *Int Stat Inst Proc* 1973;11:393–400.
66. Sedransk N. From informed consent to patient choice: a new protected interest. *Yale Law J* 1985;95:219–99.
67. Guyatt G, Sackett D, Taylor DW, Chong J, Roberts R, Pugsley S. Determining optimal therapy — randomised controls in invividual patients. *N Engl J Med* 1986;314:889–92.

68. Kratchwell TR, ed. *Single subject research: strategies for evaluating change.* Orlando: Academic Press, 1978.
69. Barlow DH, Herson M. *Single case experimental designs: strategies for studying behaviour change.* New York: Pergamon Press, 1984.
70. Sacks HS, Berrier J, Reitman D, Ancona-Berk VA, Chalmers TC. Meta-analysis of randomised controlled trials. *N Engl J Med* 1987;316:150–5.

Amyotrophic Lateral Sclerosis,
edited by F. Clifford Rose.
Demos Publications, New York © 1990.

21

Computer Simulation of Motor Neuron Disease: Its Implications for Therapeutic Trials

G. Kuether and H.-G. Lipinski

Neurologische Klinik der Technischen Universität, München, F.R.G.

Motor neuron disease (MND) is a degenerative disorder of the voluntary motor system, leading to a progressive loss of motor neurons in the spinal cord, the lower brain stem, and the motor cortex. Due to the degeneration of alpha motor neurons, an increasing number of muscle fibers become denervated, and muscular weakness and atrophy develop.

The etiology and pathogenesis of MND still remain obscure. Despite numerous therapeutic trials with a large variety of agents, no efficient therapy has been found. Although real therapeutic effects on the progression of the disease have never been observed, there exists a clear idea of what beneficial effects should look like. *Causal* therapy is characterized by a direct action on diseased motor neurons; its interference with the pathological process will result in either complete stoppage or slowing of neuronal death. Clinically, this will lead to a stabilization or decreased deterioration of muscle force. *Symptomatic* therapy will leave the underlying disease process unaltered, but may delay or slow the development of weakness by an improvement of compensatory mechanisms, which occur naturally in the motor system. An increase of reinnervation capacity, as attempted by the administration of gangliosides, is such a mechanism (1,2).

For the patient and physician, the deterioration rate of muscular force and the spread of pareses describe the progression of the disease process. Consequently, the quantification of muscle force is a central element of all protocols designed for the evaluation of therapeutic effects (1–8). A basic assumption of this approach is that there exists a relationship between the number of motor neurons lost and the amount of weakness. In mathematical terms, this relation may have certain characteristic features: The relation may be one to one, which means that to each number of lost motor neurons a concrete value of force decline can be assigned. If there is proportionality between both parameters, then the death of a larger number of motor neurons will result in a corresponding larger decline of force. In this case, a linear function describes the relationship, and the loss of a certain number of motor neurons will lead to a constant decline of force, irrespective of the stage of the process (i.e., the number of surviving motor neurons). Only on this condition will an exact description of the development of weakness be sufficient to determine the time course of motor neuronal death.

There are some lines of evidence suggesting that the relationship between the number of lost neurons and the amount of weakness is not linear. Electromyography (EMG) as well as muscle histology show that denervation of muscle fibers in MND is continuously accompanied by reinnervation (9–15). Its intensity may show large variability in different patients. This reinnervation process leads to an increase in the size of the remaining motor units. If there is a corresponding increase of the force generated by these units, reinnervation may compensate for the loss of motor neurons at least to some extent. Under this assumption, the number of lost neurons will not always correlate with the decline of force.

It is likely that these effects are most pronounced at the beginning of denervation, when sufficient intact motor neurons are available. Toward the end of the degenerative process, reinnervation will lead to quite opposite effects. With increasing motor-unit size, the loss of an individual unit will contribute to a larger amount of weakness when compared with the onset. For interpretation of the clinical course of MND and the evaluation of therapeutic effects, it is essential to have more than such a qualitative description. For instance, a trial may be planned for the test of an agent intended to increase the sprouting rate, so that we would need to estimate the effect an enhancement of reinnervation exerts on the development of muscular weakness. Other questions arise such as: What is the number of surviving motor neurons at a given stage of the disease? Are there situations conceivable in which an efficient therapeutic agent cannot lead to observable changes in the clinical course of the disease? To answer these questions, the relationships between motor neuron decay, sprouting rate, and preservation of force should be known.

Unfortunately, experimental analysis of these complex interactions is extremely limited. In MND patients, we can study only the changes of those parameters (such as muscle force) indirectly related to the disease process. Exact values for some essential factors (such as the sprouting rate) are unknown (16). Furthermore, even if values of all parameters in a given patient were known, this would be a fixed combination and would not describe their mutual interdependence. For a detailed study it would be necessary to manipulate single parameters to observe the effects any variation has on the course of the disease.

If an object under study does not allow a direct experimental approach, a theoretical model based on mathematical formulae may allow further insight. Such a theoretical analysis has two distinctive approaches: (a) The first attempts to describe the elementary processes of the system by using mathematical tools such as differential equations. Their solution would describe the behavior of the entire system. Although this is the customary way of analyzing natural processes, there are some disadvantages with this method that restrict its use. It is often virtually impossible to find an exact solution to a differential equation, so that the result can be obtained only approximately. Furthermore, the use of differential equations requires that the described parameters are consistent. In addition, the solution of a differential equation may be ambiguous because it provides coefficients the biological meaning of which is not clear from the onset, and this necessitates further interpretation. (b) The second approach has advantages when probing the problem of motor neuron degeneration. Here, only some elementary rules governing the behavior of the components of the system (i.e., motor units) need to be defined, e.g., their structural properties (motor-unit size, number of motor units) and the sprouting rate determined. The complex process of neuron loss with concomitant denervation and reinnervation of muscle fibers is subject to a stochastic program, called Monte Carlo simulation. Before starting the calculation, an arbitrary time course for motor neuron decay is chosen. The sequence of neurons that are lost will be determined by a random generator. Thus, the complexity of the system's behavior needs no deterministic description because it has been modeled by the stochastic process itself.

The model we present here is confined to the simulation of a pure lower motor neuron lesion. The programs were written in FORTRAN IV and were run on a DEC LSI 11/73 computer. In this chapter we have given a short description of some of the obtained results relevant to the evaluation of therapeutic trials in MND. A detailed report will be given elsewhere.

THE MODEL

The computer model used in our studies has some similarity to a model independently developed by Cohen and co-workers for the analysis of histological alterations occurring in denervated muscle (17). For the simulation of the degenerative process the representation of two sets of elements is necessary (18): (a) the set of muscle fibers and (b) the set of motor neurons that innervate it. Each motor neuron innervates a certain number of muscle fibers which together form the motor unit. The fibers of a single unit are spread over a certain area of the entire muscle. The number of motor units, their size, and the territory they occupy can be varied within a large range. During the running of the simulation program the number of surviving motor neurons and the number of innervated muscle fibers are continuously registered

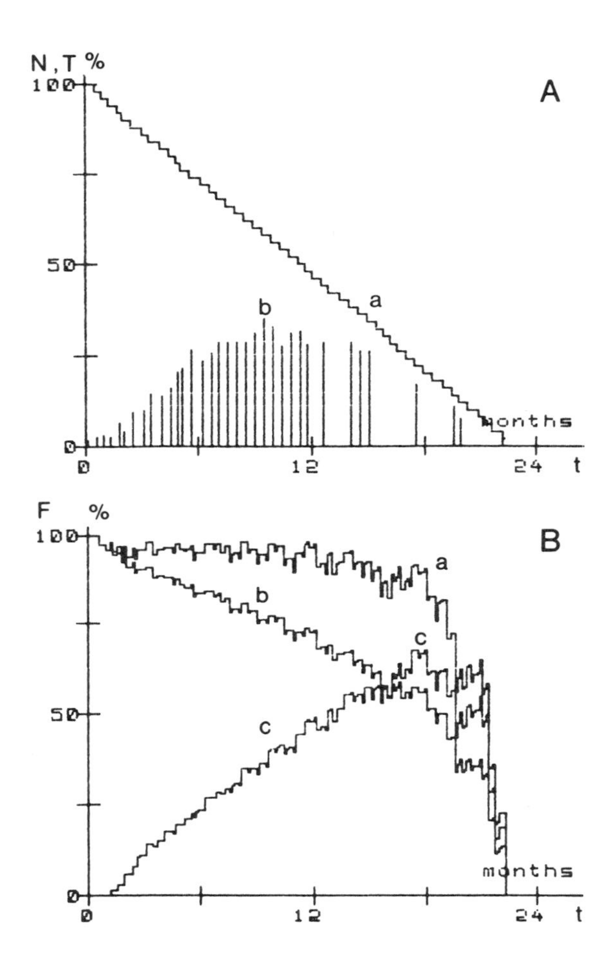

FIG. 21-1. Simulation of motor neuron degeneration with a linear decay. Duration of the process was 22 months, sprouting rate was 60 μm/month, decentric overlap of motor units. There were 49 neurons and 9,604 muscle fibers. **A**: Curve a — Number (*N*) of surviving neurons (in percent); *t* = time; Curve b — Vertical bars inside the diagram: prolongation of muscular force decline (T) in percent of the total process duration. **B:** Curve a — Simultaneous recording of the total number of innervated muscle fibers (F) in percent; *t* = time. This curve describes muscular force, if a force factor=1.0 is assumed. Curve b — Assumed muscular force with force factor = 0.5. Curve c — Percentage of reinnervated muscle fibers.

graphically on a monitor. Their decline describes the simulated degenerative process. The death of an individual motor neuron is represented by its elimination from further simulations. Because of subsequent denervation of its muscle fibers, the total number of innervated fibers declines.

Reinnervation results in new contacts being established between denervated fibers and surviving outgrowing motor axons. Given a concrete sprouting rate, a subprogram searches for denervated muscle fibers in the neighborhood of innervated muscle fibers. Each innervated fiber is thought to be the starting point for outgrowing axons, thereby simulating terminal sprouting. The sprouting rate, and the distance between intact axons and denervated fibers, determine the time before new contacts have been established. This reinnervation leads to an increase in the total number of innervated muscle fibers. Due to the effects of sprouting, surviving motor units increase in size. To study the influence that the time course of motor neuron loss has on the actual number of innervated muscle fibers, arbitrary types of motor neuron decay can be determined before the calculation is started.

Figure 21-1 gives an example of a program run describing typical features of the performed calculations. In the upper diagram, the time course of motor neuron decay is registered (Fig. 21-1A, curve a). We considered the degeneration of 49 motor neurons that innervated a total of ~10,000 muscle fibers. Thus, the motor unit size was approximately 200. An individual unit covered an area of one-tenth of the entire muscle with a mean overlap of 20 motor units. In the lower diagram (Fig. 21-1B), curve (a) represents the total number of innervated fibers. This is the sum of those muscle fibers that are in contact with their original motor neurons, plus those fibers that after denervation received axonal sprouts form surviving neurons. If we assume that the force generated by these innervated fibers is proportional to their total number, then curve (a) in Fig. 21-1B is a representation of the decline of muscular force. However, denervated muscle fibers atrophy, and hence the force they generate decreases. To assess these changes, a further coefficient could be introduced into the calculations by determining the proportion of generated force in respect to the initial value ("force factor," ranging from 0 to 1). For instance, a force factor of 0.5 indicates that reinnervated muscle fibers generated 50% of their original force (Fig. 21-1B, curve b).

To estimate the intensity of axonal sprouting, the percentage of reinnervated muscle fibers is continuously registered (Fig. 21-1B, curve c). The efficiency of reinnervation can be expressed in different ways, e.g., by looking at the time t for the difference between the number of innervated fibers with and without reinnervation. This would give a measure for the efficiency of sprouting. An equivalent method was used in our calculations. Efficient sprouting has the effect that the total number of innervated fibers declines to a certain value of time Δt later with, than without, reinnervation. This delay may also represent the clinical effect of reinnervation. Concrete values are given in the vertical bars in Fig. 21-1A, curve b.

Curve (a) in Fig. 21-1A describes the decay of motor neurons as well as the total number of innervated fibers if no sprouting occurs (force factor = 0). Comparing (a) in Fig. 21-1A with curve (a) in Fig. 21-1B, we find a considerable distortion due to the effects of sprouting. No direct relationship exists between

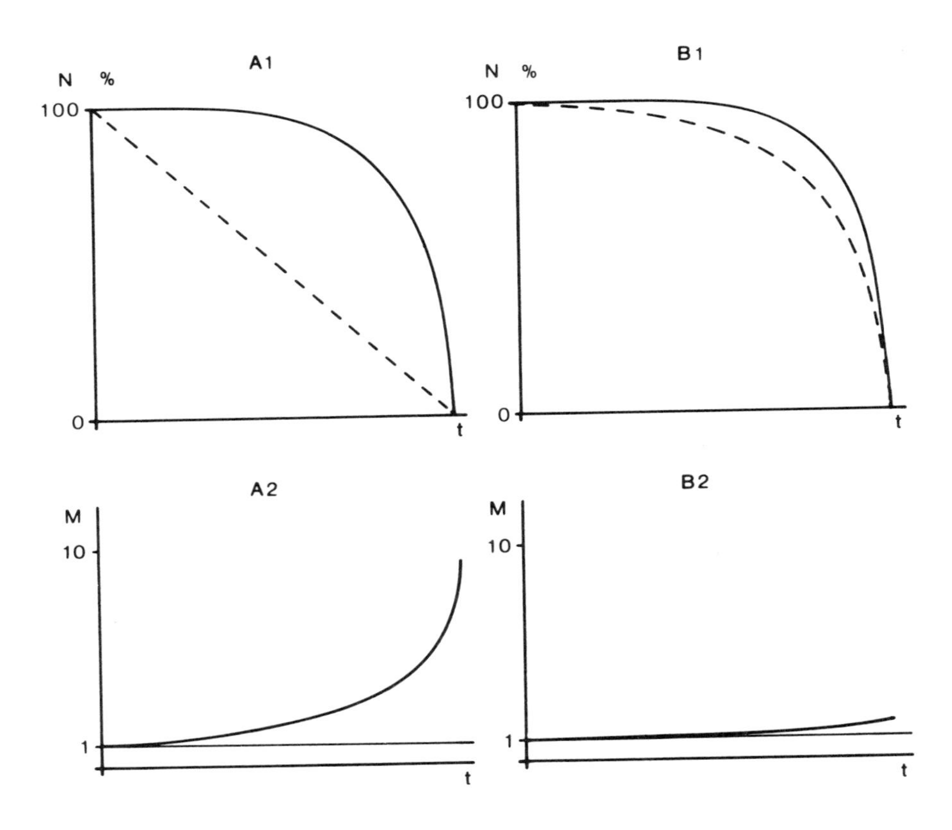

FIG. 21-2. Simulation of motor neuron degeneration with a linear (**A**) and accelerated (**B**) decay; smoothed curves. Process duration was 22 months, sprouting rate was 60 µm/month. There were 49 neurons, and 9604 muscle fibers. A1, B1: Broken line represents decay of motor neurons (*N*) in percent; continuous line indicates number of innervated muscle fibers or muscle force with force factor = 1.0. A2, B2: Increase of the mean motor unit size (*M*) in relation to the original value; *t* = time.

the number of surviving neurons and the amount of preserved force, which confirms our previous qualitative description. In the initial stages of the disease process there is a good compensation for lost motor neurons by efficient sprouting. In this phase, continuous loss of neurons is immediately compensated for by outgrowing axons, as visualized by the steep increase in the percentage of reinnervated fibers (Fig. 21-1B, curve c). Thus the initial compensation of motor neuron loss by sprouting may conceal death of motor neurons, so that the onset of paresis need not coincide with the beginning of the disease process. If we have patients with preceding effective reinnervation and generalized, although slight, weakness, this may be too far an advanced stage of the disease process and not suitable for therapeutic trials.

Depending on the time course of motor neuron decay and the effects of reinnervation, variable resultant curves may be obtained (18). In contrast, our calculations showed that identical resultant curves may be due to quite distinct processes (Fig. 21-2). In Fig. 21-2A1 and 21-2B1, two identical resultant curves are shown, but the underlying processes of degeneration and reinnervation we assumed were quite distinct. In Fig. 21-2A1, a linear decline of motor neurons with efficient reinnervation was assumed. In Fig. 21-2B1 we see an accelerated decay of motor neurons without relevant reinnervation. It is obvious that the initial conditions for a therapeutic trial are quite different. With linear decay there is a good compensation of the initial loss of motor neurons. Muscle force starts to decline when a considerable number of all motor neurons have already died. Fifty percent of the original force is preserved with only ~10% of all motor neurons left. In contrast, curve B1 in Fig. 21-2 was obtained by assuming an accelerated decay without relevant sprouting effects. In this case, the percentages of surviving motor neurons and preserved muscular force show a close relation. At any stage of the disease causal therapy would find more intact motor neurons.

Is it possible to distinguish the two processes in human patients? Both processes are characterized by different effects of reinnervation, as reflected by different changes in surviving motor units. In the first case with efficient sprouting, motor-unit size continuously increases (Fig. 21-2, curve A2). In the second case, only minor alterations in the remaining motor units will be found (Fig. 21-2, curve B2). EMG or muscle biopsy offer the opportunity to differentiate between the two processes, so that, by using EMG methods changes in the motor-unit potentials can be detected and compared with the decline of muscular force.

All these considerations apply to a disease process that is strictly confined to the alpha motor neurons in the lower brain stem or spinal cord, thereby modeling progressive bulbar palsy or spinal muscular atrophy. Because ALS is characterized by a combined degeneration of lower and upper motor neurons, what happens if we assume an additional involvement of the upper motor neurons? Does this change the dynamics of the process and its clinical manifestation? To date, no satisfactory model is available that simulates this disease under realistic conditions, due to our incomplete knowledge of the anatomical and neurophysiological features of this system and the complexity of a program needed to make calculations. Our discussion, therefore, is restricted to some principal considerations of an extremely simplified system. Here, an individual upper motor neuron shall be connected to only one lower motor neuron, and the impulses of the upper motor neuron are assumed to be sufficient to activate the corresponding lower motor neuron.

If this lower motor neuron degenerates, denervation and reinnervation occur as described above (Fig. 21-3a). Quite another situation will be found if the degenerative process starts in the upper motor neuron (Fig. 21-3b), because its corresponding lower motor neuron cannot be activated, and force

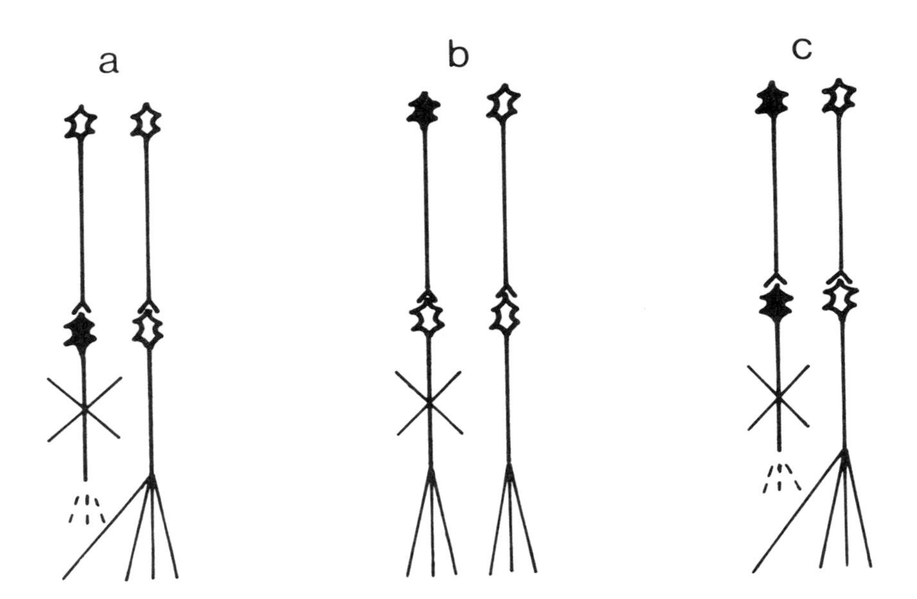

FIG. 21-3. Combined lower and upper motor neuron degeneration (black symbols for the soma indicate degeneration). **a**: Pure lower motor neuron loss with collateral reinnervation. **b**: Onset of degeneration in the upper motor neuron, no excitation of the corresponding lower motor neuron. **c**: Additional loss of the corresponding lower motor neuron, now with beginning collateral reinnervation.

will decline. In contrast to a lower motor neuron lesion, the muscle fibers remain innervated and no reinnervation can take place. If no central sprouting occurs, no regaining of force can be expected. In a subsequent step, this inactive lower motor neuron may die (Fig. 21-3c); its loss will not increase the paresis of the muscle. Instead, its fibers will become denervated and thereby available to reinnervation with a consecutive increase in force.

It is obvious that, even in this simplified system, the affection of both upper and lower motor neurons will introduce new dynamic properties that depend on the location of degeneration and its sequence. If the architecture of the system is modeled in a more complex manner, with converging and diverging synaptic contacts, considerable alterations in the behavior of this assembly during the degenerative process can be expected. This deserves further investigation. However, even these crude qualitative descriptions illustrate how difficult it may be to deduce the time course of neuron degeneration from the development of weakness.

DISCUSSION

The present investigation shows that some basic properties of the complex process of motor neuron degeneration with denervation and reinnervation of muscle fibers can be analyzed by using a computer simulation program. Its advantage is the free variability of the incorporated parameters, which allows a detailed study of their mutual interdependence. Furthermore, such a theoretical approach compels a more precise definition of terms which otherwise would retain their inaccurate meaning, e.g., "efficiency" of reinnervation had to be described in terms of our model, and we could determine some factors by which it is influenced (i.e., sprouting rate, stage of the disease).

The computer model at the present stage of development can only be considered a simplified description of natural processes occurring in human disease. We used only a crude description for muscular force, which assumed proportionality between the number of innervated muscle fibers and the amount of generated force. No distinction was made between fiber types and the different forms of muscular contraction. Despite these restrictions, there are some fundamental principles that have to be considered in clinical studies of the disease. In our model, efficient reinnervation has been shown to cause considerable discrepancies between changes of clinical parameters such as muscular force and the loss of motor neurons. In corroboration with experimental results, our theoretical analysis showed that up to 50% of all motor neurons may be lost before marked weakness develops (9,19,20).

Clearly, these results introduce new aspects to the discussion of therapeutic trials in MND. As pointed out earlier, the large variability of the natural course of the disease explains the difficulties in ascertaining therapeutic effects (21). Due to inappropriate composition of treatment and control groups, false-positive or false-negative results may arise.

Our computer simulation indicated that even identical clinical courses of the disease may be due to quite distinct underlying pathomechanisms that offer different initial conditions for the detection of beneficial effects. Depending on the efficiency of reinnervation, the percentage of intact neurons may vary to a large extent even at similar stages of muscular weakness. It may be asked why it is so essential to find a certain amount of intact neurons at the beginning of therapy. Intact neurons of healthy subjects have a certain life expectancy. In mathematical terms, for each neuron there exists a concrete probability of dying within a subsequent time interval. A degenerative disease process can be described as an additional increase in this probability. In contrast, the effect of a causal treatment can be expressed as a reduction of this increased likelihood of subsequent death. The concrete value of the resulting difference depends on the activity of the degenerative process and the potency of the administered agent. If we describe the efficiency of a therapy in these probabilistic terms, then we expect the occurrence of beneficial effects to depend on the number of available neurons. The more motor neurons that are alive at the beginning of therapy the better are the chances of achieving therapeutic effects.

There is another reason that underlines the importance of the initial number of motor neurons for the outcome of a trial. It seems unlikely that a therapeutic agent will exert its effects instantaneously after first administration. Due to its pharmacological properties some time is needed to cross the blood–brain barrier, to reach affected neurons, and to assume the local concentration necessary for therapeutic effect. Furthermore, some time may elapse until the agent changes the pathological alterations inside the cells. In the meantime, depending on the progression rate of the disease process, more motor neurons will die. If the initial number of intact neurons is too low, no effects will be observed despite the potency of the administered agent to influence the disease process.

For these reasons, a rational planning of therapeutic trials has to separate favorable clinical courses of the disease from less favorable ones. For instance, patients in too-advanced stages of the disease will have no chance to obtain protection from further neuronal degeneration, if the few remaining neurons have begun irreversible changes in their metabolism. Other patients with efficient antecedent reinnervation cannot be expected to show a pronounced response to therapies that improve sprouting; with their natural reinnervation capacity they may already have reached an optimum of compensation. Due to efficient sprouting their number of intact nerve cells will be low even in the initial stages of the disease, and clinical assessments will underestimate the severity of the disease. Furthermore, in these patients the final deterioration rate has to be considered to be a direct consequence of preceding reinnervation rather than to be the result of an accelerated motor neuron death.

This leads to the problem of adequate selection criteria which should enable differentiation between distinct types of the disease process. Up to the present, there has been a tendency to increase criteria for admittance to therapeutic trials in ALS, because of the absence of laboratory markers that could unequivocally determine the diagnosis. Because this depends largely on the clinical examination, the diagnosis can be established only after there has been progression of the disease with spread of muscular weakness, so that other disorders can be excluded. This means that the lower limits for entry into trial are shifted toward advanced stages of the disease. Considering our model calculations, a fundamental dilemma arises: The more the diagnosis is certain, the more is known about the time course of the disease, the lower the number of available motor neurons, and thus the likelihood of achieving beneficial effects. Vice versa, with a higher number of intact neurons, the chance of exerting therapeutic effects is increased. However, at the same time, uncertainty about the further development of the disease is increased, so that it is more difficult to ascertain these effects. Therefore, to some extent, uncertainty will remain, irrespectively of the choice of selection criteria.

The problem is to minimize these sources of error by using sensitive and applicable methods for assessment of the initial stages of the disease. With quantitative force measurements, the onset of paresis may be detected long before clinical symptoms arise (5,8). Because reinnervation has been shown to be a determinant factor in the clinical course of the disease, its longitudinal study should contribute to a better evaluation of trials in MND. With diverse EMG methods (conventional EMG, single-fiber EMG, macro-EMG) it is possible to quantify the alterations of motor units due to denervation and reinnervation (11–13). Correlation of these findings with quantitative force measurements would allow an estimation of the efficiency of axonal sprouting, so that EMG recordings of representative muscle should accompany quantitative force measurements.

The considerations illustrate the difficulties of conducting and interpreting therapeutic trials in ALS. With available methods of assessment caution is required in assessing any therapeutic effect on the degenerative process itself, not least because a change in the time course of muscular weakness may have several reasons, many of them not directly related to motor neuron loss. The appropriate clinical and statistical methods measure only an alteration in the clinical course of the disease. If positive effects can be achieved, further investigations are necessary to substantiate a direct action of the used agent on the pathological process within the motor neurons.

In conclusion, there are two different levels at which therapeutic effects can be evaluated. The first is of phenomenalogical nature, describing the occurrence of changes in the progression rate of the disease, irrespective of its origin, an aspect of utmost importance to patients who ask for alleviation of their symptoms. At a second level, the investigator has to analyze the obtained results, to look for possible sources of false-positive or false-negative effects, and to decide whether an enlarged trial is necessary to confirm the results. This is perhaps the most delicate part of ALS research because its results influence both the studies of other clinical investigators and the expectations of patients. By advancing this form of theoretical analysis it may help in finding improved methods for therapeutic trials, and so avoid erroneous conclusions in the search for efficient therapies.

Acknowledgment: We thank Dr. J. Hetet for helpful discussions. This study was supported by the Stifterverband für die Deutsche Wissenschaft, ZE 170/7BY, and the Wilhelm Sander Stiftung, 87.021.1.

REFERENCES

1. Bradley WG, Hedlund W, Cooper C, et al. A double-blind controlled trial of bovine brain gangliosides in amyotrophic lateral sclerosis. *Neurology* 1984;34:1079–82.
2. Harrington H, Hallet M, Tyler HR, Ganglioside therapy for amyotrophic lateral sclerosis: A double-blind controlled trial. *Neurology* 1984;34:1083–5.

3. Mitsumoto H, Salgado ED, Negroski D, et al. Amyotrophic lateral sclerosis: effects of acute intravenous and chronic subcutaneous administration of thyrotropin-releasing hormone in controlled trials. *Neurology* 1986;36:152–9.
4. Kelemen J, Hedlund W, Orlin JB, Berkman EM, Munsat TL, Plasmapheresis with immunosuppression in amyotrophic lateral sclerosis. *Arch Neurol* 1983;40:752–3.
5. Andres PL, Hedlund W, Finison L, Conlon T, Felmus M, Munsat TL, Quantitative motor assessment in amyotrophic lateral sclerosis. *Neurology* 1986;36:937–13.
6. Andres PL, Finison L, Conlon T, Thibodeau L, Munsat TL, Use of composite scores (megascores) to measure deficit in amyotrophic lateral sclerosis. *Neurology* 1988;38:405–8.
7. Munsat TL, Andres PL, Finison L, Conlon T, Thidodeau L. The natural history of motor neuron loss in amyotrophic lateral sclerosis. *Neurology* 1988;38:409–13.
8. Kuether G, Struppler A, Lipinski HG, Therapeutic trials in ALS — the design of a protocol. In: Cosi V, Kato AC, Parlette W, Pinelli P, Poloni M, eds. Amyotrophic lateral sclerosis. New York: Plenum, 1987:265–76.
9. Hansen S, Ballantyne JP. A quantitative electrophysiological study of motor neuron disease. *J Neurol Neurosurg Psychiatry* 1978;41:773–83.
10. Erminio F, Buchthal F, Rosenfalk F. Motor unit territory and muscle fiber concentration in paresis due to peripheral nerve injury and anterior horn cell involvement. *Neurology* 1959;9:657–71.
11. Stalberg E. Electrophysiological studies of reinnervation in amyotrophic lateral sclerosis. In: Rowland LP, ed. *Human motor neuron diseases.* New York: Raven Press, 1982:47–57. (*Advances in Neurology*; vol 36.)
12. Stalberg E, Sanders DB, The motor unit in amyotrophic lateral sclerosis studied with different neurophysiological techniques. In: Rose FC, ed. *Research progress in motor neuron disease.* London: Pitman, 1987:105–21.
13. Swash M, Schwartz MS. A longitudinal study of changes in motor units in motor neuron disease. *J Neurol Sci* 1982;56:185–97.
14. Coers C, Telerman-Toppet N, Gerard JM. Terminal innervation ratio in neuromuscular disease. *Arch Neurol* 1973;29:215–22.
15. Lester JM, Silber DI, Cohen MH, Hirsch RP, Bradley WG, Brenner JF. The co-dispersion index for the measurement of fiber type distribution patterns. *Muscle Nerve* 1983;6:581–7.
16. Bradley WG. Recent views on amyotrophic lateral sclerosis with emphasis on electrophysiological studies. *Muscle Nerve* 1987;10:490–502.
17. Cohen MH, Lester JM, Bradley WG, Brenner JF, Hirsch RP, Silber DI, Ziegelmiller D. A computer model of denervation-reinnervation in skeletal muscle. *Muscle Nerve* 1987;10:826–36.
18. Kuether G, Lipinski HG. Computer simulation of neuron degeneration in motor neuron disease. In Tsubaki T, Yase Y, eds. *Amyotrophic lateral sclerosis — recent advances in research and treatment*, Amsterdam, New York, Oxford: Excerpta Medica, 1988:131–8.
19. McComas AJ, Sica REP, Campbell MJ, Upton ARM. Functional compensation in partially denervated muscles. *J Neurol Neurosurg Psychiatry* 1971;34:453–60.
20. Sharrard WJW. Correlation between changes in the spinal cord and muscle paralysis in poliomyelitis. *Proc R Soc Med* 1953;46:346–9.
21. Brooke MH, Fenichel GM, Griggs RC, et al. Clinical investigation in Duchenne dystrophy: 2. Determination of the "power" of therapeutic trials based on the natural history. *Muscle Nerve* 1983;6:91–103.

Subject Index

D

Q

R

Notes